# THE WAY TO

# NATURAL BEAUTY

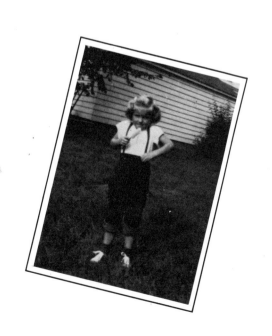

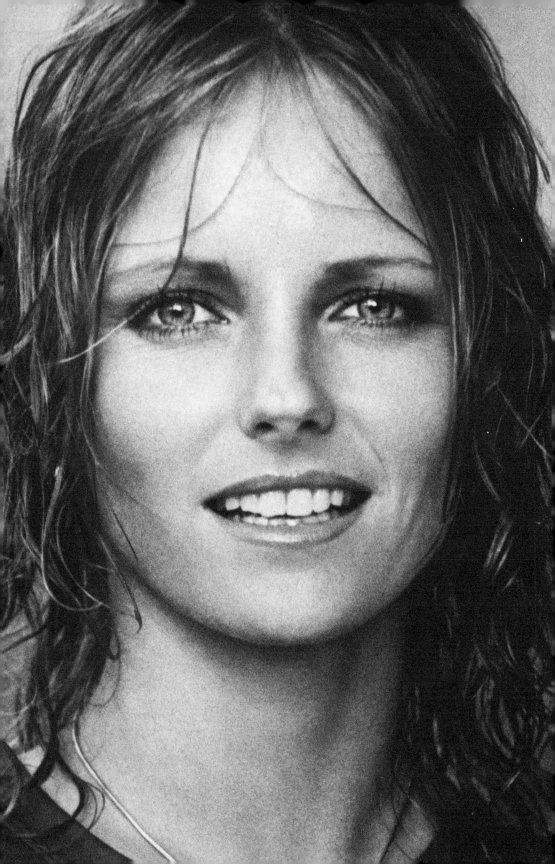

# Cheryl Tiegs

## THE WAY TO NATURAL BEAUTY

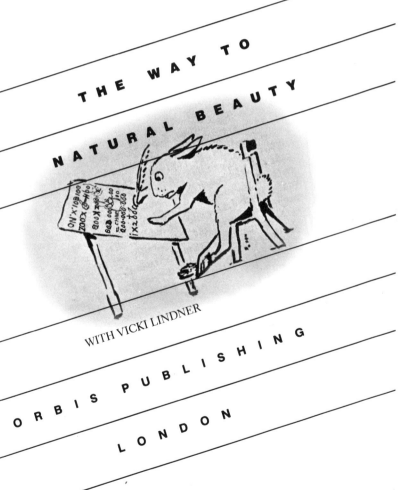

WITH VICKI LINDNER

ORBIS PUBLISHING

LONDON

The quotation on page 36 comes from "Not Waving but Drowning," in Selected Poems of Stevie
Smith. Copyright © 1964 by Stevie Smith. Reprinted by permission of New Directions.
The quotation on page 132 comes from A Separate Peace by John Knowles.
Copyright © 1960 by Macmillan, Inc. Reprinted by permission of Curtis Brown, Ltd.
The quotation on page 171 comes from Snow Country, by Yasunari Kawabata,
translated by Edward G. Seidensticker. Copyright © 1956 by Alfred A. Knopf, Inc.
Reprinted by permission of the publisher.
The quotation on page 172 comes from Snakes and Ladders by Dirk Bogarde.
Copyright © 1978 by Holt, Rinehart & Winston.
The quotation on page 284 comes from "Adam's Curse," in Collected Poems of
William Butler Yeats. New York, Macmillan, 1956.

Grateful acknowledgment is made to:

The Condé Nast Publications Inc. for permission to reproduce six photos from
VOGUE, thirty-six from GLAMOUR, three from BRIDE'S, Copyright © each year, 1963
through 1979, by The Condé Nast Publications Inc. All rights reserved.
The Condé Nast Publications LTD. for permission to reproduce two photos from
British VOGUE. Copyright © each year, 1963 through 1979, by The Condé Nast
Publications LTD.
Bernard Leser Publications PTY, LTD. for permission to reproduce two photos from
VOGUE AUSTRALIA. Copyright © each year, 1963 through 1979, by Bernard Leser
Publications PTY, LTD.
The Hearst Corporation for permission to reproduce fifteen photos from HARPER'S
BAZAAR, and two from GOOD HOUSEKEEPING. Copyright © The Hearst Corporation
1968 through 1980.
Additional picture credits appear on page 288.

FOR MY PARENTS

AND

FOR STAN

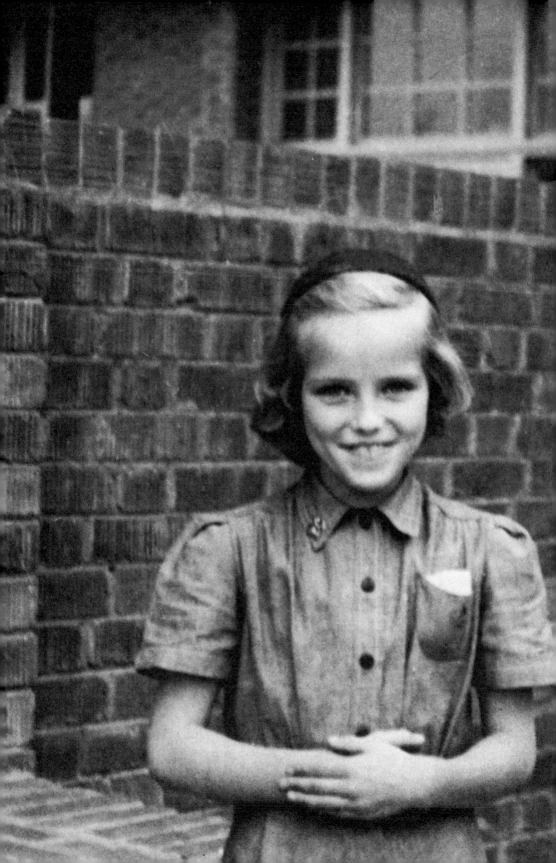

# Contents

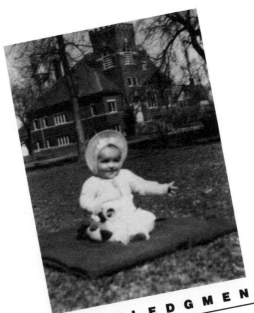

# ACKNOWLEDGMENTS

I would like to thank my best friend Christy for the original idea; Peter Beard for his enthusiasm, inspiration and photography; Barbara Shapiro for her patience and good cheer; Marvin Israel for the look of the book; Russell Goldsmith for years of creative counsel; Ray Cave for being a believer; Tony Mazzola for his help from the beginning; Michael Korda of Simon & Schuster; Charles Schulz; Bill Connors; Bill King; Ellen Bernie; Paula Greif; Mary Giatas; Phil Pessoni; Betty Thompkins; Gary Simmons; and Jack of Kenneth's Salon.

I am grateful to my friend Steven Aronson for his crisp editorial overview; and to my sister Vernette, for always being there.

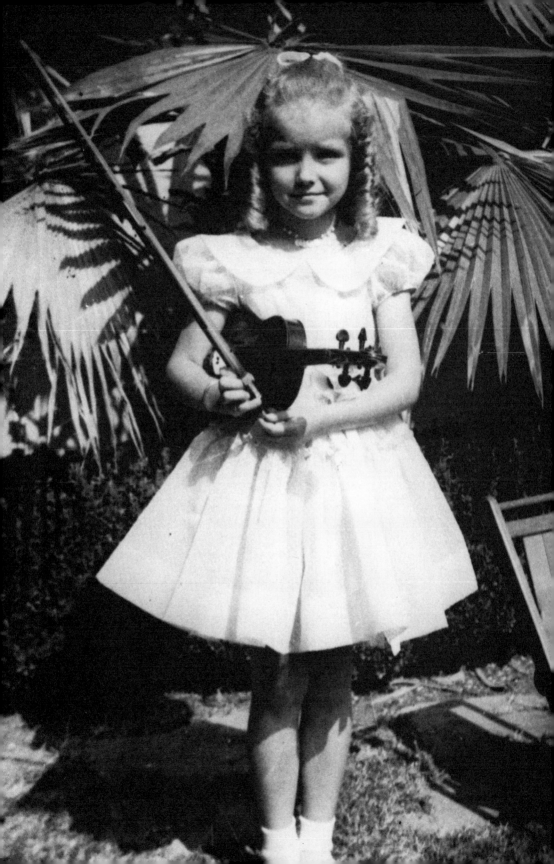

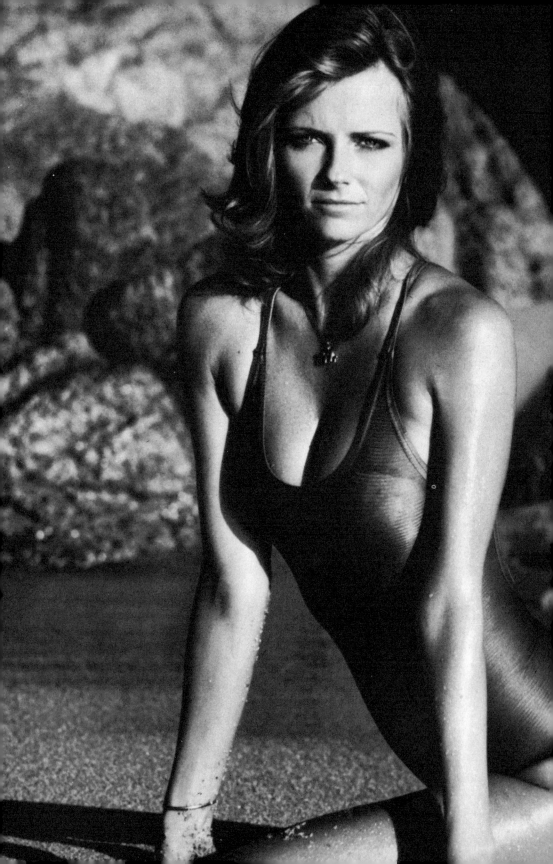

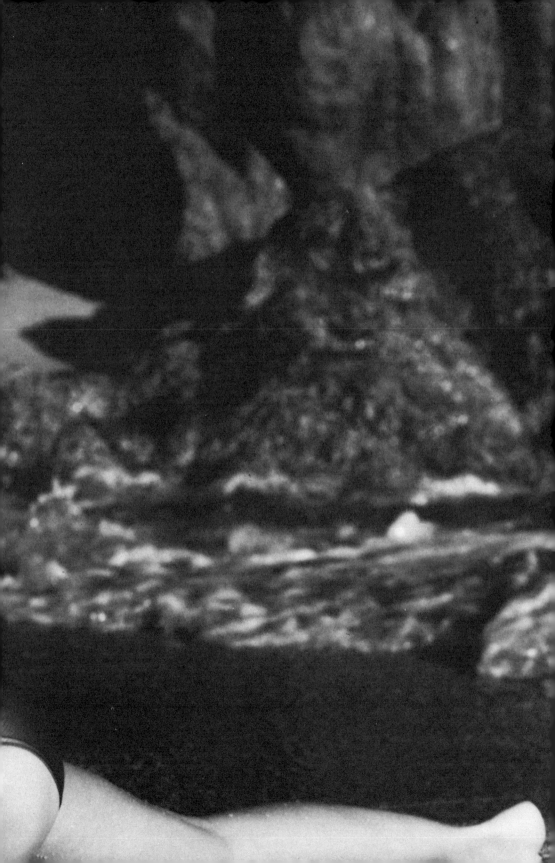

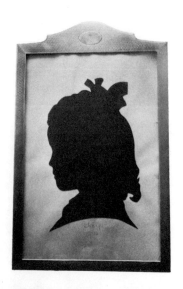

# A "Natural Beauty" Who Me?

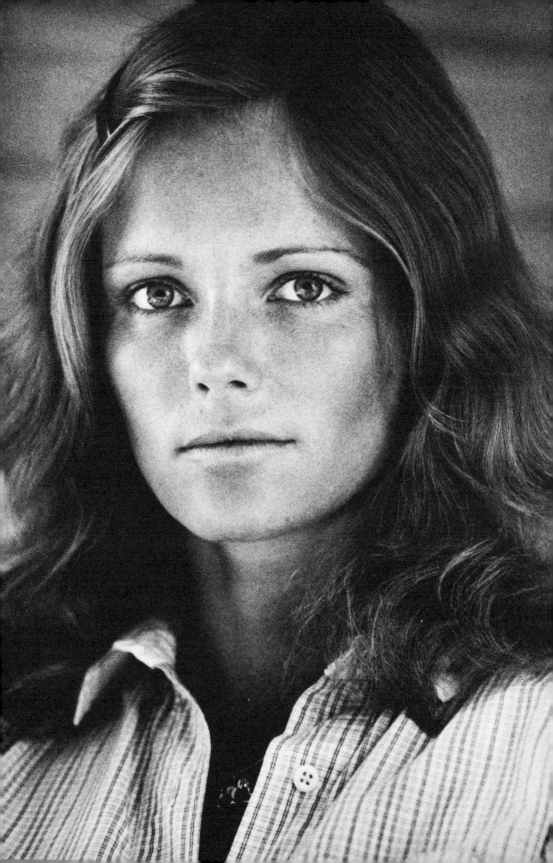

can't count the number of times I've heard or seen myself described in print as a "Natural Beauty." And every time, I think to myself, "They should only know what it takes to be 'Naturally Beautiful.' " The term conjures up a woman who has been born beautiful and who, without any effort at all, remains beautiful. Well, there's no such creature in life—there never was, and there never will be.

Famous models are often thought to be possessed of some kind of magic—fortunate, gorgeous, remote creatures, strangers to blemishes and telltale wrinkles, circles under the eyes, extra pounds, blasted "cellulite," bulging thighs, and such mundane worries as which shoes to wear with which dress and whether or not a certain dress is smart or out of date. All a model has to do is enlist the hired help of a famous hair stylist or makeup artist to put the final touch, the coronet of perfection, on her inborn glamour and aside from that, she never has to fret over her appearance the way other women do—right?

Wrong. A thousand times wrong. Twenty push-ups, fifty sit-ups, and one hundred leg raises a day wrong.

So people think I look the way I do because I'm "lucky," because, like Beatrice in *Much Ado*, I was "born under a star that danced." When I work out at the gym, for instance, many of the women there come up and ask me, "What in the world are *you* doing here?" Or else they don't say anything and just sneak looks at me to see how I do the exercises. Or else they can't look at me at all! (The implication being that exercise is strictly for that accursed race: the overweight and out of shape.)

What was Cheryl Tiegs doing there? Listen my children and you shall hear. . . . At the beginning of my modeling career I ate my way up to a gross 155 pounds; I had a double chin (*two* double chins), and when I lay down I couldn't find my hipbones, and I was only twenty. My egregious eating habits almost destroyed not only my figure but my skin, and no ad in the lost and found was going to get my hipbones back. I had made the near fatal mistake of believing that I *was* a "Natural Beauty" and of taking my looks—my slim figure and good skin—totally for granted. But I was caught in that mistake—by Nature, which was there to remind me, quickly and unsparingly, that the gate-

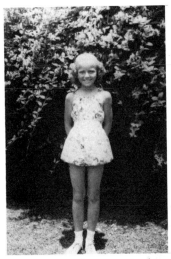

*Minnesota ~ 1955.*

way to good looks is good health, plain and simple. I should say plain but *not* so simple, because I had to be remade, to remake myself, to start over again at the beginning: I had to study nutrition to learn what foods would keep me slender without depleting my energy. And, reflecting one day on my reflection in the mirror, I determined to learn how to exercise, so I could get my shape back *and keep it*. No makeup artist, no hair stylist in the world, no cosmetician, can supply a woman with the essentials of beauty: a good figure, good skin, and eyes and hair that shine (Oh, these magicians can see to it that she glitters for an evening, but then the glitter fades like fairy gold). The essentials are *her* job—*your* job, *my* job—and, as I was to discover, it requires self-discipline, knowledge, and a heavy bundle of work.

When I went into modeling, I was like any other girl just starting out—insecure. When you're that young, you think that everyone else is super-confident about themselves and that you're the only one who's weak in the knees and a little white about the lips. What I didn't realize is that there's a side to insecurity called vulnerability and it's very sympathetic, at least at the moment when a person is on the verge of accepting full responsibility for herself. It's true that love and even admiration can be killed dead by cockiness. My point is that there's more than one kind of self-assurance just as there's more than one kind of vanity and more than one kind of love.

In those days, I knew next to nothing about fashion. I didn't have a clue about how to style my hair—I don't even think they had hot rollers back then—or about how to apply makeup. (I remember sneaking into the gym in high school and putting on mascara, which we were forbidden to wear till we turned sweet sixteen, putting it on illicitly in front of the mirrors with all the other girls—it was almost as wicked as running off to the bathroom to smoke. My sixteenth birthday present was a tube of lipstick—baby pink, what else? I can almost taste it now. I had that tube of lipstick for a whole year, I had so little occasion to use it. But it made me feel quite the little lady. As for mascara, my first time out I went and did a really stupid thing—I got it in my hair. One of my girlfriends said, "What's that in your hair?" I ran to the bathroom, feeling I'd touched the rock bottom of the sea. She hadn't even noticed my lush lashes that I'd used the mascara to accentuate. Anyway, those were the days.) I didn't know the first thing about putting a "look"

together or anything about the tricks of our trade: perfumes, accessories, shampoos, skin-care products. I
was very fortunate to be working with the top makeup
artists and hair stylists and they gave me advice, for
which I was extremely grateful (at times their advice
amounted to a life line). But I also had to learn for and
by myself just when their advice was not for me. I had
to find—by trial and error, hit and miss—the look that
expressed *my* personality, that made *me* feel comfortable with myself and that in turn attracted others to
me. My experience was not by any means unique or
exotic; in fact, if anything it was representative. Every
girl who believes in the life of her looks has to learn
the exact same things about beauty that I did.

A "Natural Beauty," then, is not some lucky girl who
can keep her looks without having to work hard at it;
nor is she a butterfly of fashion whose appearance is
contrived, self-conscious, and quite lacking in *sincer-
ity*. Natural beauty, to the extent that it can be
achieved at all, must embody a contemporary attitude
toward life, energy, incorrigible vitality, and, at one
and the same time, self-awareness and a wholly delightful forgetfulness of self. No so-called natural anything would dream of erecting a wall of artifice
between herself and her beholder—such as wigs, excess makeup, the falsest of false eyelashes, untouchable bouffants teased into man-o'-war hair helmets, and
ferociously flamboyant clothes; if she resorts to *any* of
these things, she won't stay "natural" for long, will
she? Some women can manage an elaborate facade
better than others; occasionally it even becomes the
hallmark of their style, but sooner or later this artificial
look comes unglued, and then the big picture drops
out along with the frame.

I usually feel too made-up after a single modeling
assignment. My feeling is my makeup's had its brief
heyday before the cameras, and I can't wait to get
home and wash it all off. Too much makeup has the
air of a premeditated device and the look of a barrier,
and a barrier is a bar or obstacle, something that re-
strains or obstructs or limits access—in this case to
none other than y-o-u. You should want other people
to feel as if they could touch you. A natural look, the
look that should be coveted, lets you and others relax
and communicate.

Not that a natural look should be *so* laid back, so
once-over-lightly, that it's drab and eminently ignor-
able. Too little attention paid to hair, makeup, and
wardrobe, too little awareness of and sense of style,

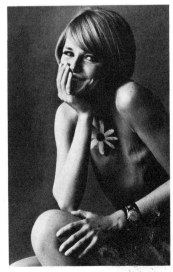

e NOON
BC for
n footage
no + ck charge
E PB
Xmas shop
d. Ave
s to look....
LD —
for Xmas
decorations
for bath
5:00
arrives
d with

le toe
etta's
th Ribbon
books
c. etc.
D
corated

Barbara
or
oj + Vodka

on Nix.....
emory of
who ran

her way
Wyeth")
B.
le HERD

HOME
rvice:
hysoisse, steak tartar, etc, etc.

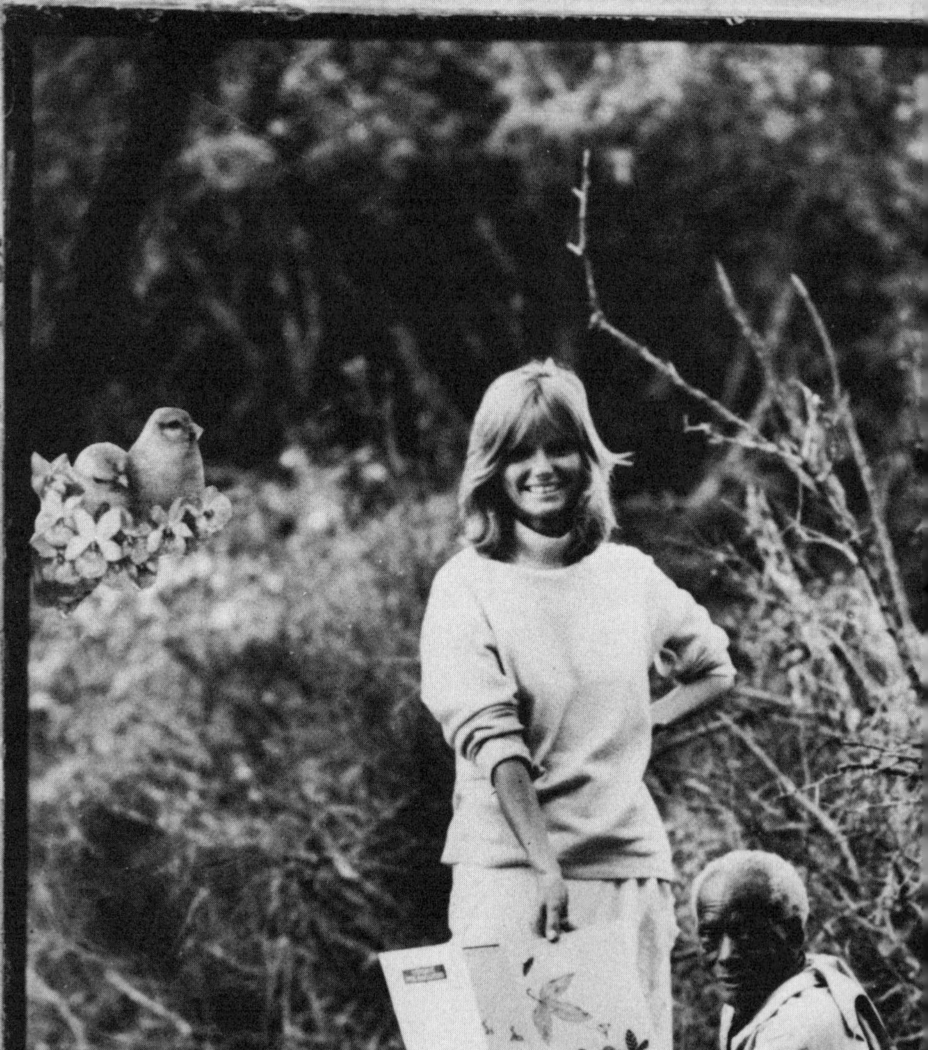

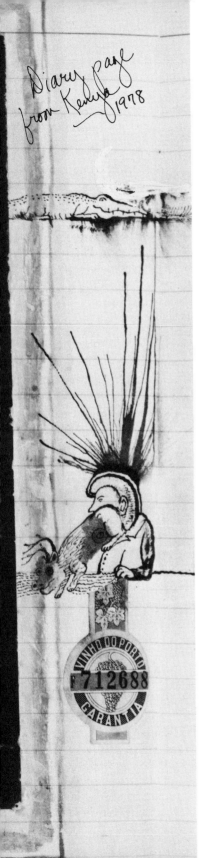

will definitely not advance the good fortunes of a woman. The modern beauty industry has provided us with so many aids that there is no reason for any woman's doubts about her physical appearance to remain unanswered. Today every woman can look her best, and none of us need actually see the work that went into the enterprise. Vanity can be innocent of trivial or corrosive self-regard; it can be healthy, positive—"I am proud of who it is I am! I deserve some attention and I hope I get it!" The dictionary opposite for "vain" is "useful," but vanity can be a very useful quality. All of us, to one degree or another, are vain. And so we should be. Let us, then, contrive to be vain of our good figures and fine clothes.

The natural look, once you know how to bring it off, should take relatively little of your time. I hate spending even an hour fussing in front of a mirror in the morning, and even if I didn't mind it as much as I do, my schedule doesn't permit it. (Whose does these days? Nothing could be more alien to the spirit of our times than spending most of one's spare moments working on your face and body and thinking about the way you look; the world today makes wider claims on all of us.) And yet, an attractive appearance is always going to help make a woman more effective in both her career and her personal life—not least of all by giving her the self-confidence she needs. But if she becomes obsessed with being and staying attractive, if that becomes the sole focus of her life and she works ceaselessly and unremittingly at it, it may pay her back by consuming her at the expense of her spontaneity and spirit.

During the two years at the beginning of the seventies, when I took "early retirement" from modeling, I went into a decline. The most glaring manifestation of this decline was that I was spending much too much time on my appearance, scrutinizing every infinitesimal wrinkle and pore and examining my hair twenty times a day for split ends—I'd clearly lost all perspective. At the age of twenty-two, there I was anticipating and dreading the signs of old age. The narcissistic impulse that we are all born with and that, with a little luck, fades into the background around about puberty, was reasserting itself—but in a sadly disproportionate way. When I returned to work, however, I began consorting again with my active, unself-regarding self—there were so many things to do, so many places to go every day that the unhealthy concern over my appearance just phased itself out. And do you know something? I looked much the better for it. I was once more focusing on the worthwhile things, and though achieving and maintaining good looks was still important to me (and a major part of my work as well), I was doing it with far less pettiness and drudgery.

Now once again I found that there was joy to be had in preparing myself for a special evening—a leisurely bath, a facial, a little experimentation with a glittery new makeup, and the *pièce de résistance*—the selection of some fabulous outfit to wear. I was doing it again with great *désinvolture*, offhandedness. Before these special occasions I enjoy toying with new makeup products, hair colorings, conditioners, and other gadgetry. But the rest of the time I want my beauty regimen to be convenient and easy to accomplish.

Every woman needs and wants a system of health and grooming habits that will both insure she'll look her best most of the time and also take as little as possible of her time. No woman need feel "desperate" about her appearance every time she's faced with an important event in her social or professional life. Good looks are looks that wear well—they don't disintegrate under pressure. But they do require maintenance; the woman who cultivates her physical qualities instead of nagging at and worrying over them will never "suddenly" discover that she is fifteen pounds overweight or that her hair is a dull, drab mass or mess or that her skin is dry or that she has nothing stylish in her wardrobe. She's learned the basics of a good appearance, and the first basic is that she must conscientiously follow an everyday regimen, including a low-calorie, nutritious diet, exercise, and a program of skin care to keep her figure and skin in good, humming condition. Just add to this a good haircut, a well-thought-out wardrobe, and a practical selection of cosmetics, and her most elegant self will always be available to her.

No system should be rigid, it should always leave room for the growth and change and experimentation that are so important to a contemporary look.

Experiments, however, must be undertaken with some caution and mitigated by self-knowledge. Once, during my fallow housewife period, I was going to a theater première in Los Angeles and I wanted to look special, so I took a long silk scarf and swirled it around my head a few times and knotted it in a fanciful way and let it droop. When I presented myself to my husband, he suggested as politely as possible under the

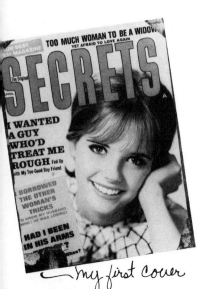

*my first cover*

dire circumstances that maybe I didn't *need* that special creative touch. I undid the wild scarf, and went out to meet the world on my own terms, posing as nobody but myself. And that's who I've remained.

The chapters that follow are full of tips (many of them drawn from the professionals I've worked with for so long) for health and beauty that I've learned in my fourteen years of modeling and my thirty-two years of living. Reading them should help you come up with a look that expresses your personality and attracts others to you. I'm going to ask you a lot of questions about yourself and if you take the time and trouble to answer them honestly, I think you'll be able to pick out the areas where you need help the most.

Throughout the book I'll be coming back again and again to the crucial relationship between the body and the mind. How you think and feel is related in a thousand ways to how you look. I'll be suggesting methods for you to enhance your positive points and make light of, or disguise, your less good ones—by means of regular exercise, carefully applied makeup, and practical wardrobe selection. The time-saving things I've learned to do throughout the day to maintain my appearance in the face of a murderously busy schedule, you'll learn to do, too. And, to give the complete picture, there's a list of the most common mistakes women make when it comes to diet, exercise, makeup, skin care, and wardrobe.

It is no unattainable ideal to which I would have you aspire. It's your own originality that I hope to help you find—an active, healthy attitude. I want you to cultivate or develop your own humor and sympathy. The rest is icing on a really good cake.

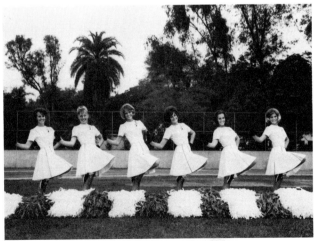

— the wave of the future ...

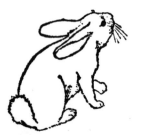

# 1

# Just Starting Out

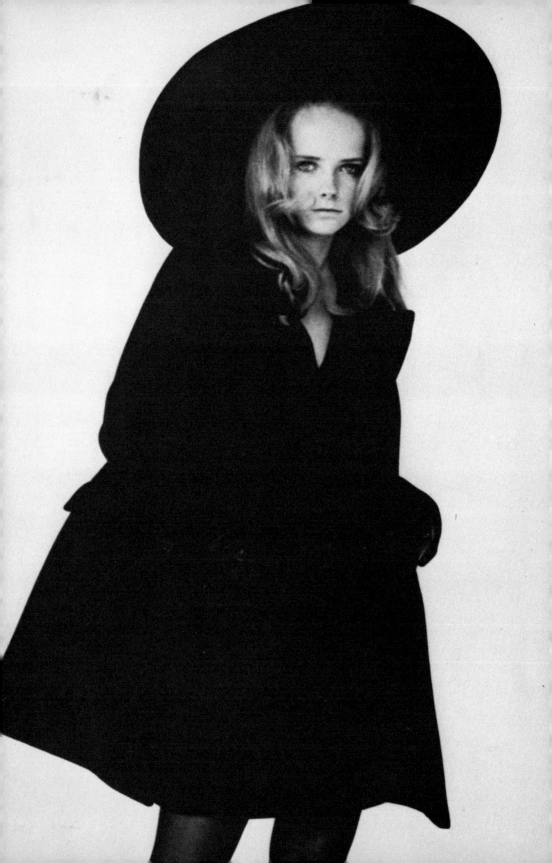

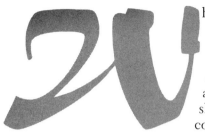hen I was a teen-
ager in Alhambra,
California, my
best friend was
always running
across the street to
show me her latest
copies of *Seventeen*
and *Glamour*. "Cheryl," she would say, "you should
be a model!" And I thought that she must see something in my round face and tall, skinny body that I
couldn't see. I took in what she was saying, but I didn't
believe it.

I studied the faces of the beauties in those magazines as if they were lessons I had to learn for school
—Jean Shrimpton, Colleen Corby, Twiggy. I remember some of the individual pictures—the perfect pro-
files, pixie noses, lustrous, long, beautiful hair, and
snazzy clothes. I wanted so badly to order a neat plastic raincoat in one of the photo spreads; it was the
most weightless adornment I had ever seen, and underneath it there was a heavenly blue sweater and a
deep blue skirt. Luckily I didn't have the money. I say
luckily because the coat just wouldn't have looked
right on me—for one thing, I didn't have the wardrobe to wear underneath all that see-through plastic.
The world of the models in all those photo spreads
seemed about as unattainable as that raincoat. I
planned to go on to college and become a teacher or
a nurse.

But then a representative from a modeling agency
came to speak to a girls' club at my high school; he
talked about the experience and meaning of being a
model, from every perspective, and he brought the
modeling world a little closer—at least it ceased to
belong simply to the province of the magazines. After
his talk, he took three or four of us aside and invited
us to come to Pasadena for an interview.

I remember I put on a little pink dress—with a pink
bow on top of my hair—and my mother and I went up
to his office. He accepted me on the spot as a student
in his modeling class—along with a thousand other
girls, as I would discover—for a fee of three hundred
dollars. We were given lessons in etiquette by a woman
who would always enter the classroom in white gloves
and tell us things like to be sure and eat our ice cream
at dinner parties before it melted; and there were lessons in commercials conducted by a woman who had
never done a commercial but who would hold up an

eraser with the greatest authority and show us how to say meaningfully, "this is the *best* eraser"—and we believed her.

I modeled in department store fashion shows for free, and occasionally I would get up at dawn and report as an extra for *Beach Blanket Bingo*-type movies for twenty-five dollars a day (once, I was cut from the final picture because I didn't have enough "personality"; you were supposed to dance wildly, with complete abandon—I guess they wanted a real bimbo and I wasn't it). So many times my mother and I would drive in for interviews after school and they'd say "thanks but no thanks, you're beautiful, but don't call *us*." Sometimes I posed for snapshots to be used by illustrators of fictional magazine stories; for this I received the princely sum of five dollars an hour. On one occasion I modeled at a nursing home; I paraded around in the fashions I'd brought with me, and I chatted with each and every patient. The patients would then judge me on my "charm, personality, and fashion appeal" —which seems kind of funny, when I think about it now. The head of the modeling school always encouraged us to try out for contests like "Miss Army" and "Miss Navy." My best friend in the school won Miss Navy and I was one of the runners-up. I remember the little army hats—honest-to-God official ones— that they'd stick on you if you placed. Who voted I don't remember. I actually won one of those contests once; for a few hours I got to hold the awe-inspiring title of "Miss Rocket Tower." Somebody'd needed a girl to get up at five in the morning and go to the beach and stand by a rocket tower. It was in the papers and that was it, that was the end of my reign.

Meanwhile, some of the other girls had been talking to other modeling agencies, and I began to get the drift that ours was the smallest of small-time. It was about then that I made the switch to the Nina Blanchard agency, and that's when my career—if you'll forgive the rocket tower imagery—really took off.

I was determined from the start to work as hard as I could and to go as far as hard work could take me. This often entailed giving up social functions or even just being quietly with my friends. I found myself rushing to modeling interviews right after school. I had to go to a lot more interviews than I care to remember before landing a single job. My hair wasn't long enough, I was too tall—there were at least a million things wrong with me, but everyone was very nice— what they said, in effect, was "Don't give up."

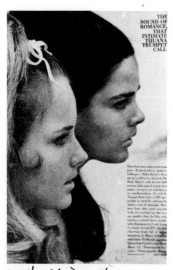

with ali MacGraw in St. Thomas

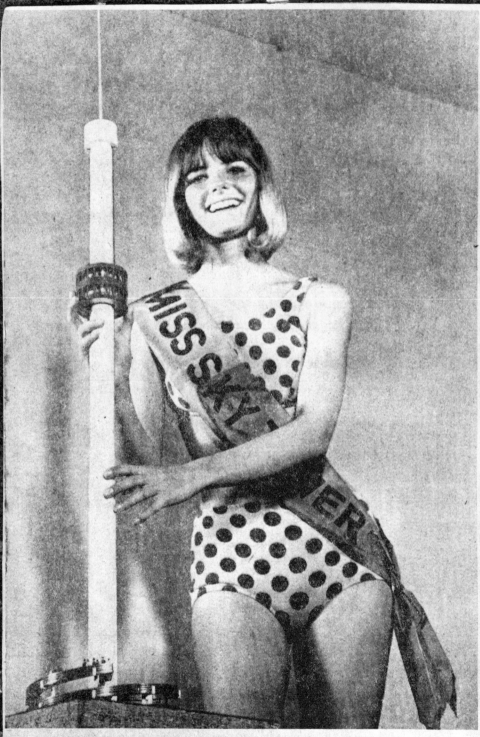

**MARINELAND SKY TOWER** — Model Cheryl Tiegs shows model of new California landmark under construction at Marineland of the Pacific. The Swiss - built tower is scheduled to be opened by July 4. Taller than the Statue of Liberty, it is equipped with a two - tier rotating elevator that will whisk visitors skyward for a panoramic view. Sixty persons can ride at a time, 30 to each tier.

My family and friends supported me in my career choice, although my father was always uneasy about the "types" he was afraid I would meet in the fashion world. "Of course you can model," he told me, "but I'd feel better if you didn't date anybody in the business." Naturally, within a month I disobeyed him. I dated a very cute male model who took to wearing boots with two-inch heels because he was shorter than I was. My father had very little to fear; my date from the wild, wicked world of modeling would always take me to the local donut shop after the movies—it was all very innocent, really.

When I was seventeen I entered California State College in Los Angeles, planning to major in English. I continued modeling on the side. My big break came when I was featured in a Cole of California bathing suit ad, a dreamed-of double-page spread, that appeared in national magazines. The fashion editor of *Glamour*, Julie Britt, saw me in the ad and booked me sight unseen to model *Glamour*'s spring fashions for a week in St. Thomas in the Virgin Islands. Julie's call had come at four, and the flight to St. Thomas was at seven. I was half in shock as I packed, and I did what you do when you pack half in shock—I packed all the wrong things: it was winter in L.A., so I took care to

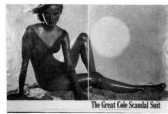

— the Cole Scandal

The Great Cole Scandal Suit

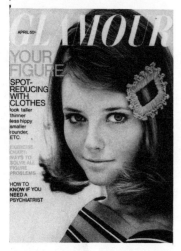

include all my little wool dresses and I forgot to bring my bathing suit. The other model on the trip was Ali MacGraw; we shared a room, and that first night she unpacked all these beautiful summer dresses from Paraphernalia. She kept apologizing for having so many. When she got an eyeful of what I'd brought with me, she threw me a dress across the room and said, with thoughtfulness and tact I'll never forget, "Maybe you'd like to try something like this?" I'd never seen clothes like Ali's. In Pasadena you didn't have Paraphernalia. For the first time ever, I felt I looked really fabulous: I had on the latest, hottest little numbers, and don't forget, I was in the tropics. (Would St. Thomas ever be the same?)

This assignment resulted in my first *Glamour* cover, and then *Glamour* started booking me regularly. Usually they came out to California and photographed me there, but once they flew me to Fort Lauderdale during Easter when the college kids were there *en masse* for their vacation (talk about density!)—the famous hairdresser Kenneth was along and he introduced me to the more sophisticated look of big fat braids down my back. And I got to go to New York several times. During all this, I was still very much the college English major, but frankly, it's the real world that's always taught me the most.

I knew that for any aspiring model, New York was the place, the "Big Time," the ultimate challenge, and that in order to "make it" I would have to make it there; New York was the one and only place to be validated, or at least the one and only place where the validating counted. I decided to try my luck there. With a model friend from California, Kelly Harmon, I moved into a suite on the first floor of the Shoreham Hotel on West Fifty-fifth Street just off Fifth Avenue. Every morning at four the garbage was collected right in front of our windows, and that included the discarded bottles from the Shoreham restaurant. It was all a little much for Kelly and after about a month she moved back to L.A. I was on my own now.

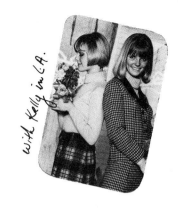

with Kelly in L.A.

I didn't understand the labyrinthine bus and subway systems, so getting myself to job interviews was a real ordeal, weighted down as I was with a heavy shoulder bag full of hairpieces, falls, makeup, hot rollers, lingerie, and other atrocities as well as my newly purchased appointment book. It was August, and the heat was coming down out of the sky and up out of the pavements, annihilating whatever was foolhardy enough to be in between them; by the end of a day like that, I was drained and limp, and my feet had blisters.

And whenever I felt confident that I had conquered the bus system, my uptown bus would turn a corner on me long before my stop and I'd have to get off and start all over again—that is, if I'd been lucky and been observant enough to notice in time.

One shooting that summer was scheduled for Bridgehampton in the outer reaches of Long Island. Our first stop was Cartier's where we picked up thousands of dollars' worth of jewelry, which was to be our lavish and light-hearted companion on the trip out. So far so good. But then it began to pour, and then, an hour out of New York we had a flat tire. The fashion editor swerved over to the right lane and told me to stay in the car with the Cartier family jewels while she went to get help. Presently she reappeared with a tow truck in hand or rather, in tow. And soon we were on our way again. By the time we arrived at this beautifully restored old barn, it seemed a true haven. And suddenly I just felt that things were going to work out for me.

Thanks to the exposure I'd had in *Glamour*, I was booked fairly solid from the beginning. I accepted every job I was offered except lingerie, which I didn't think was dignified.

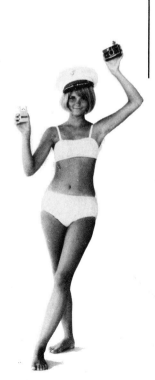

"Big Time" in N.Y.C.

Aside from lingerie, though, there was practically nothing I didn't model. I modeled for newspaper advertisements, women's magazines, catalogs, you name it. I had as many as five bookings in a single day. Often on a job they ask you to work "just a little overtime," so then you're late for the next place, and you have to work "just a little overtime" there to make up for it—so it's a bit of a vicious circle till you arrive home late at night, practically good for nothing but sleep.

I soon discovered that those etiquette classes at the modeling school back home weren't going to come in all that handy and that if I let the ice cream melt at a dinner party in New York, the harlequin sky wouldn't fall in. I watched how the other models did their hair. I knew next to nothing about the high-fashion look. I remember Lauren Hutton patiently sitting in the studio—she'd just finished putting her makeup on and now she was taking the trouble to show me how to put mine on. I had always admired her. She was just beginning to make it really big with *Vogue* covers. That day, when she went out in front of the cameras, she looked *incredibly* sexy—she kind of pushed her breasts up. Then I went out, feeling like a little girl with lots of makeup on but, thanks to Lauren, looking pretty good. I've always found that the top models are the most helpful as well as the most down-to-earth.

Many of my first assignments were for modeling junior fashions. I must say I rarely met an unpleasant client or editor, and I never encountered the legendary lecherous photographer who chases models around the studio and worse.

Particularly wearing on my nerves were the "go-sees" or tryouts, where there were usually ten or twenty girls waiting to be called for their interviews for a given commercial. These were sometimes referred to as "cattle-calls," a cruel but accurate word for them. One day I saw a girl I particularly looked up to come out and I thought, well, that's that, she'll get the job, and the next day when I was told that in fact *I* was the one who'd gotten it, I realized the quick turnover there could be.

Modeling is a mercurial profession as well as a very demanding one. Yesterday's sensation is today's has-been. Also, modeling, like everything else in life, can be lonely. The girls are young; usually it's the first time in their lives they've been alone in a big city, and they're making unrealistic amounts of money to boot. They are criticized by some clients; glorified, even apotheosized by others. I don't need to tell you that

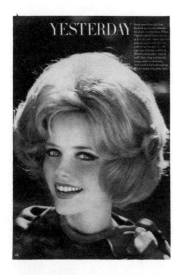

this can be confusing psychologically, and it's not hard to lose perspective. There was one beautiful but temperamental girl who burst into tears—for no reason I could ever fathom—at every shooting. I went on a trip with her to Hawaii with Helmut Newton for *Vogue*, and every single day she cried. If she didn't like how she'd been made up, she would go into the bathroom and wipe off the makeup and throw it at the mirror or something equally insulting to the makeup artist, who would then have to start all over. In Hawaii you have these tropical showers for half an hour every so often —they're no big deal, but every time we had one, she would go stalking off somewhere to cry. At first everyone had quite naturally sympathized with her, but by the end of the trip nobody but nobody was speaking to her. It was clearly only a matter of time before clients and photographers were going to refuse to accommodate her. There are just too many lovely young girls —emotionally stable ones—competing for the same jobs. I considered myself lucky to be a model. I was grateful for the opportunity to make so much money per hour, and I wanted to give the clients what they were paying for—not only efficiently but as graciously as I could manage. I made it my policy to be businesslike and, once I got the gist of the bus and subway systems, prompt.

Julie Britt, Barbara Stone (my first New York agent), and many of the photographers and magazine editors I had worked with helped me adjust to New York, whose ways are wonderful but also sometimes very mysterious. They helped me move into empty, cold apartments—I had about seven apartments in one year, I think. I finally found one I really liked, on Seventy-second Street between Second and Third avenues—a nice brownstone. I was working so hard I didn't have time to furnish it, but a photographer I knew brought over a table and some chairs he had, and on Christmas day, with my apartment as "spacious and sparse as an autumn wood," another photographer friend appeared at my door with a tree, so I would at least have the smell of Christmas.

And Julie Britt would make sure I got out of the city from time to time. She invited me to her weekend house in Water Mill on Long Island where, with the sea on one side and the potato fields stretching, it seems, into infinity on the other, I always had the somehow comforting feeling of being at land's end. So little by little I got used to New York. I'll say one thing for it: never for a moment was it boring.

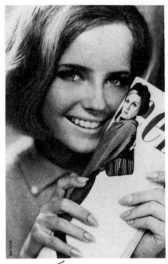

Twiggy + me...

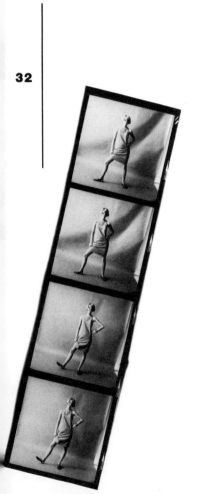

I discovered that most of the top models had never even gone to modeling school but had learned what models need to know the same way I had learned it—through practical experience and through a careful examination of the clothes, makeup, and hairstyles featured in the fashion magazines. One of the first things I noticed was how much these styles changed within a single issue even, and I realized that the most interesting models were the ones I could look at page after page and they would have a different look every time, which of course is how you last as a model. I also learned to analyze the work of the well-known photographers, how they used different kinds of lighting and the different ways they liked their models to pose for them. I remember studying the way my idol Jean Shrimpton flew across a room in *Vogue* (with the uncramped confidence of a bird!). In the privacy of my own bedroom I tried to fly—like Icarus, I was prepared to try anything once!—and what I looked like was ever so hopelessly earthbound. I also admired Twiggy, and in front of my mirror I imitated *her* bird-like pose, but my feet seemed to be made of clay or something, leaving me to wonder how *they* did it. In time I came to understand that your hips and shoulders, arms, hands, and even facial expression all have to work together in a split second of camera time. With practice and knowledge, I became quite a credible flier across rooms.

Another thing I did was buy the European fashion magazines so I could study how the European models ("mannequins" they call them over there) achieved their svelte (*soignée* they call it over there) look. I was my own guinea pig, I tried everything out on myself, and sometimes it worked, and often it didn't. Because I was a model I got to see the new fashions before other people did. I developed an eye for which styles would flatter me the most, and soon I was able to put together a look that expressed my own personality and struggling sense of style. Above all, I was no longer timid. You might not be able to see anything exactly courageous in this but one day I went out and bought a bizarre antique snake ring; I was somehow sure it would look right on me, and probably the reason it did look right on me was because I felt it would. A little thing called mind over matter, I guess.

When I first came to New York, in the late sixties, models were a lot thinner and much more dramatically made-up and stylized than they are today. They wore hairpieces, falls, and three or four false eyelashes all stuck together and then, to my astonishment, *glued* to their eyelids. I loved wearing the falls—all that hair cascading down my back made me feel as if something unbelievably romantic was just about to happen to me. (Luckily, I didn't hold my breath.) But when it came to wearing the heavy makeup, I upped and rebelled. "Go back in the dressing room, Cheryl, and put on a little more," the stylists all kept telling me, but I could never bring myself to paint my face to the degree that they wanted me to. I was new and unknown and very eager to please, but I just was convinced that exaggerated heavy makeup was all wrong for me, that it would destroy rather than enhance my looks.

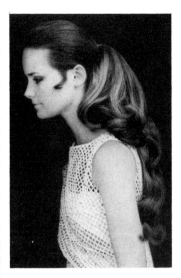

I used liner, shadow, and mascara, but I drew the proverbial line at the false eyelashes—besides making my eyes tear and itch, they gave me the queasy feeling I was assuming a false identity by masking the natural expression in my eyes. When I had them on, it was like I was wearing a hat over my eyeballs.

Then, just as my modeling career began going strong, I started putting on unwanted weight—a traumatic enough thing for anyone, to be sure, but for a model a public as well as a private event. For a long time the extra weight hardly affected my bookings. Julie Britt would just mock-groan and mock-huff and puff as she zipped me into the outfit I was to wear, and as for the stylists, they would just have to remember to order a size ten for me from the designer instead of my former size eight. But then the day came when I began bursting out of the size ten!

The stylists began having to cut my dresses and pants up the back seams to make room for my hippy hips. And the final photographs now had to be re-touched; my thighs and midriff had to be thinned down, not to mention the sum total of my two double chins. Everyone was very tactful and I shall always be grateful for their understanding during this difficult time. Barbara Stone especially, who would defend me by saying that I was "just a great big healthy California girl."

But the day of reckoning was near at hand, and like most days of reckoning it would turn out not to be without value. It was a cold, dreary day to begin with; perhaps all days of reckoning are cold, dreary days to begin with. I'd been booked by a photographer I had long admired but never before worked with. When I got to his studio, I went right into the dressing room to change. None of the clothes fit me, but I wasn't worried; I just assumed the stylists would make them

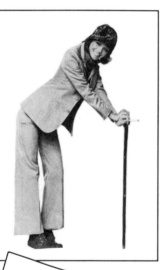

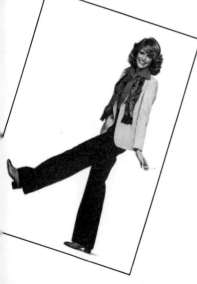

"You've come a long way, baby."

work for me, as they had always done before. But when the phone rang in the studio (what made me so agonizingly sure it would be for me?), it was my agent calling to say she'd just been called by the client, etc., etc., "Cheryl," she said, in a very embarrassed voice, "You can go home now." I gathered up my belongings with a false smile pasted to my face and left the studio, completely and utterly humiliated. Everyone there— the photographer, the other models, the stylists— knew that I was having to leave because I was just too fat for the job. The first thing I did when I got home was put on my baggy jogging suit and, in the forlorn hope of reversing reality, run around the block several times. But the second I got in the door I hit the refrigerator for a Sara Lee fix, as if fulfillment were to be found only there.

When I was twenty-two, I got married to Stan Dragoti, the brilliant "creative director" of the innovative agency Wells, Rich, Greene. We moved back to L.A., and I decided to retire from modeling—I'd worked hard in New York and I felt I needed some time for myself. Stan said, "You'll be sorry," but that's always something you have to find out for yourself—as I did, watching my self-esteem slip through the net of leisure. At first I read a great deal, took cooking lessons, tried gardening—all the sacred little tokens of domestic happiness. But, as Stan had predicted, it just wasn't enough. When people asked me how I was, I found myself talking about Stan and all the exciting things *he* was doing. I no longer had goals or any real purpose in life; soon I began to feel that I was of little or no account. But then, on a day when I had nothing more to do than peel and chop a couple of bunches of carrots for a soup, I got a call from one of my former clients asking me to consider modeling for them again. I immediately said yes, and I know that whatever the future may bring, I'll never take early retirement again.

It was during my so-called "retirement," though, that I regained my slender figure. One night Stan and I were at the movies; as usual I had one hand in the buttered popcorn and the other on a candy bar. But when a beautiful actress in a bikini appeared on the screen, the lump of dough I then was groaned inwardly, "If only *I* could look like *that* again." I was on the verge of making some Faustian pact with the devil when it occurred to me that maybe the only difference between her and me was one of will power. My fat, eating self immediately went on strike. (Well, maybe not immediately—I think I finished the buttered popcorn.) In a year of quite serious dieting I plummeted from 155 to under 120 pounds. My face and figure came back to me, but with a new maturity, my face having acquired more definition, my body more muscularity. In modeling circles I'd been known for my young, innocent look, but no more—after the trauma of these cookie-jar years (everything is the result of something, right?), my looks were at last appropriate for sophisticated, high-fashion modeling. And my exterior circumstances weren't the only thing that had changed; my whole attitude was fresher, thanks to the sheer discipline involved in exercising properly and losing weight.

Now that my "junior" days in fashion were behind me, I had access to a greater range of magazines. I traveled all over the world; I was deliciously torn in all different directions. I posed for *Sports Illustrated*, *Harper's Bazaar*, and not only for American *Vogue* but for English, French, Italian, and Australian *Vogue* as well. Some of these magazines used my name so that I began to exist a little in the public eye.

I was thrilled when the Virginia Slims people called to ask me to do a series of ads for them. I'd always thought theirs were the classiest ads. And what's more, they were going to let *me* choose the clothes I thought suited me best. For one ad I would select very sporty fisherman's gear and for another a very elegant dress that I'd wear with my hair pointing up, in the direction of the twinkling stars. When you're having a good time, the pictures turn out the best. On the night of the famous blackout in New York, I was at a friend's high-rise apartment on Gramercy Park, and I had to walk down all twenty-five flights of stairs because I was booked for a Virginia Slims ad the first thing the next morning. When I arrived at the studio, there was of course neither electricity nor running water. But there were plenty of candles and everyone was laughing and running around opening bottles of champagne. What better way to get a shooting started than with laughter and champagne? No, those were some of my best pictures.

As a lifelong sports fan, I was pleased to be asked to take part in the annual *Sports Illustrated* bathing-suit feature. We went down to Manaus, the oldest city in Brazil, to shoot. On our last day there, we went out for about two hours on a river in a canoe. I had on a thick fishnet bathing suit which I promise you the naked eye could not see through. They asked me to go

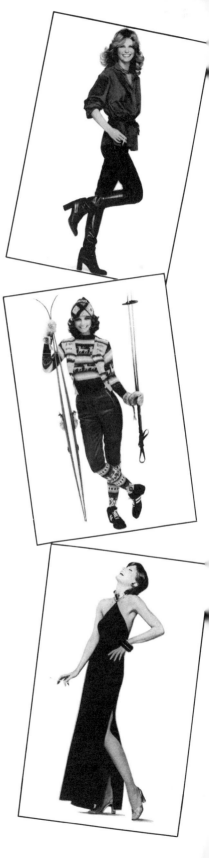

into the water, and I did. It was sunset and the water was the color of tea. When that shot was developed, you could see right through my thick suit—it must have been the combination of the light, the wetness, and the filters on the cameras. People still ask me how I feel about that fishnet bathing-suit shot. I'm not embarrassed because it was natural. I've seen plenty of photos in which the models were all covered up that were much more provocative—deliberately so. I got thousands of letters, most of them favorable, to say the least.

I was still living in Los Angeles but I was spending a lot of my time now traveling around the world. It was on these trips that I learned the difference between looking and seeing.

Travel of course has its light side, but even light sides have their dark sides. When I was asked to model a bikini in Acapulco, I accepted at once because what could be more glamorous. The photographer took me out to this huge rock in a boat, literally deposited me there like a castaway, then sped back to shore to shoot me with a telephoto lens. I noticed that the tide was rising and the rock area shrinking. Huge crabs crawled up from the waterline—closer and closer to me. I actually screamed at them, trying vainly to scare them into going back to their element. And meanwhile the water, naturally, kept rising. By now I was yelling and signaling wildly to the photographer but he either couldn't hear me or else thought I was getting all happily carried away with the job. I thought of the English poet Stevie Smith's great two-line poem, "I was much further out than you thought/And not waving but drowning." Finally the photographer got the message that his star model *was* about to be carried away—not with the job but with the tides; and rescue was at hand.

It is also possible to feel stranded in a speedboat—to this I can attest. We were on the wide, free, open seas off Honolulu; Helmut Newton, the photographer, likes the real thing, so when he discovered that we were behind an atomic submarine heading off to Alaska he was hell-bent on overtaking it. Picture me stretched out on the edge of the transom decked in white with Helmut filming all the while and me pretending I wasn't the least bit terrified I was going to be sucked into the wake of the monstrous sub. The final shot looks casual, but believe me, it was panic city all the way!

I vividly recall another colorful assignment in the tropics, where another model and I would spend hours

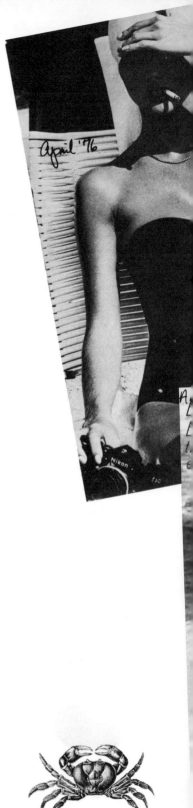

april '76

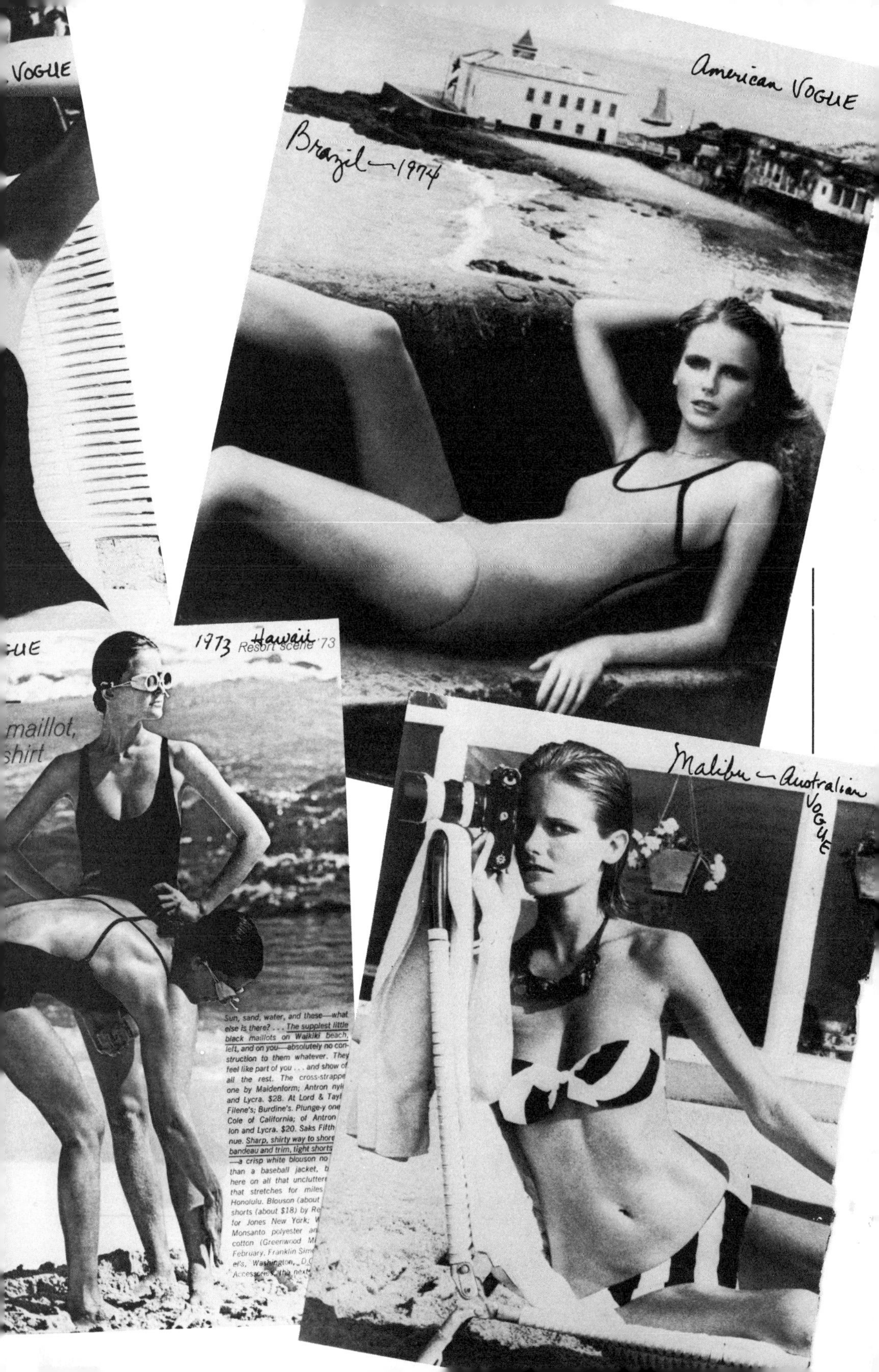

American VOGUE

Brazil—1974

1973 Hawaii
Resort scene '73

maillot,
shirt

Malibu—Australian VOGUE

Sun, sand, water, and these—what
else is there? . . . The supplest little
black maillots on Waikiki beach,
left, and on you—absolutely no construction to them whatever. They
feel like part of you . . . and show of
all the rest. The cross-strapped
one by Maidenform; Antron nyl
and Lycra. $28. At Lord & Tayl
Filene's; Burdine's. Plunge-y one
Cole of California; of Antron
lon and Lycra. $20. Saks Fifth
nue. Sharp, shirty way to shore
bandeau and trim, tight shorts
—a crisp white blouson no
than a baseball jacket, b
here on all that uncluttere
that stretches for miles
Honolulu. Blouson (about
shorts (about $18) by Re
for Jones New York; W
Monsanto polyester an
cotton (Greenwood M
February. Franklin Sime
er's, Washington, D.C
Accessories: the next

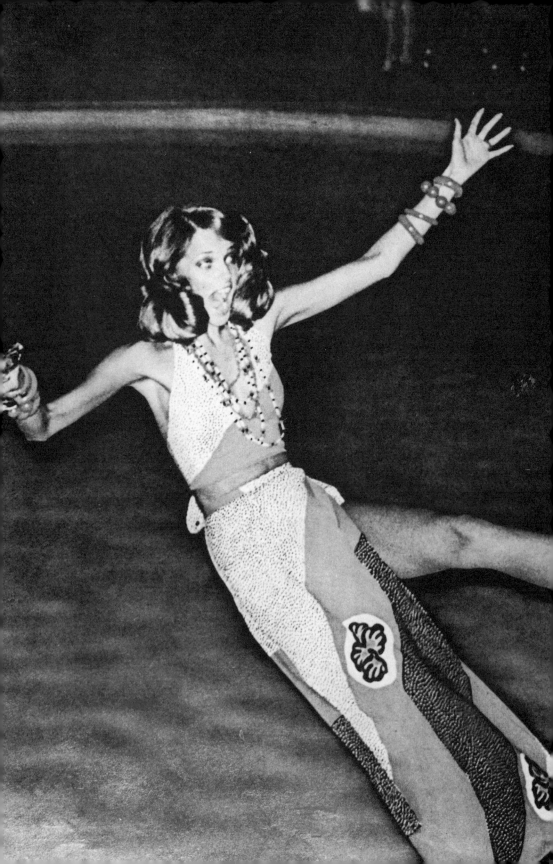

Falling for Helmut Newton.

and hours having our hair and makeup expertly done, after which we'd dress up in the most fabulous evening clothes and lay on the accessories. And *then*, dressed to the nines, we were directed to fall backwards into the pool! It took the photographer a while to get the right moment. I think we had to fall backwards into the pool twice a night for seven days running. And each time everything had to be *just right*—the champagne asparkle in our glasses, our hair, the expressions on our faces, the slits in our dresses, our shoes, necklaces, bracelets. Such was life in the higher reaches— and lower depths.

I went to Rome to model collections for Italian V*ogue*. David Bailey was the photographer. We stayed at the famous Hotel Hassler on the Piazza di Spagna —a dreamlike setting. The collections were photographed at night, so I had to work from eight in the evening till four in the morning. Around dawn, after our "workday" was over, we'd go off to some wonderful little café on the Via Veneto for eggs and champagne. It was like something out of *La Dolce Vita*. Then back I'd go to the Hassler to sleep all day. I loved having my usual schedule completed reversed for a change.

But after a while the novelty wore off and I felt like I was living out of a suitcase. I'm not saying I was a captive to my career; I don't think I was ever that. I always felt that the rewards and excitement involved in modeling were worth a little sacrifice. And anyway, for me security was not specifically synonymous with home; I had trained myself to find security wherever I happened to be (or find myself). Many models complain a lot about the stress. The amount of stress *is* great; striking poses on different continents month after month isn't all "champagne, sunglasses, and autographs." But I learned to enjoy the variety and to see the necessary travel as an often delightful extension of my inner home.

Thousands of girls have written asking me to advise them on how to embark on a modeling career. For photographic modeling, also called "print" work, there are very definite physical requirements. "Print" models are almost always taller than average (5'7" to 5'10" in bare feet), seldom weigh more than 120 pounds, and have long torsos, long legs, and long necks. Hips should measure approximately 34"–36", waist 24"–26", and bust 32"–36". They must be able to wear a size eight, the size that most fashion samples come in. Contrary to the common belief, today you can be *too* thin to model. (I have a friend who has a perfectly exquisite face, but eventually clients stopped booking her because she couldn't fill out their clothes.) Hands and feet should be shapely, skin clear, teeth white and in line, hair shining and healthy. Circles or bags under the eyes are a disqualifying feature if they're beyond the pale of the retoucher's talents.

The most important qualification for a "print" model is, naturally, a photogenic face, because it is not the model herself the client hires to advertise his product so much as it's her two-dimensional image. "Photogenic," however, does not necessarily have to mean "conventionally pretty." There are plenty of beautiful faces that happen not to photograph well, and other, more ordinary faces that do.

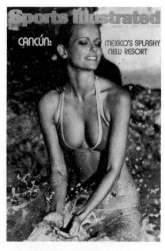

It's not possible to define the qualities of a photogenic face. Like a successful painting that can't easily be described, it could be summed up as something that—simply and mysteriously—"works." I think it's helped me to have small features, since the camera increases their size, and wide-set eyes, but there are many successful models who have large features and close-set eyes. There just aren't any rules.

For showroom, ramp and fitting models, who work for designers or fashion shows, the requirements are pretty much the same, they're just not as strict. But for any kind of modeling, the younger you start (after sixteen), the better your chances for success.

One of the most important things is to be able to work spontaneously, unself-consciously, without a morbid awareness of your every gesture and expression. This takes years of practice, of both learning and then learning how to put what you've learned into the back of your mind. This holds true for the photographer as well; he can be dragged down by techniques, filters, lenses, exposure meters—and miss the main drift of the occasion, lose his sense of its aesthetic as he pursues a more accurate f-stop. The more accomplished the model, the more naturally she will be able to work with the photographer. Some photographers operate in deadly silence like surgeons or scientists; others coax, flatter, and cajole; some work with music on; some prefer to have clients, art directors, and complex sets; others prefer to work alone and with just the bare no-scene paper. Flexibility is essential.

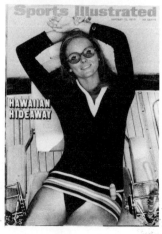

Beauty, youth, and a photogenic quality, however, do not automatically make for a successful model. Success comes with learning such things as changing hair and makeup to match the clothes you're wearing, and projecting a personality to suit the mood of the photograph. You must be able to put on a dress you don't even especially like and make it look like it was made for you, like you were just on this earth to wear it. I was lucky: most of the clothes I modeled were gorgeous, but there were times when I had to invent a way to make them appealing. A laugh can help—or an amusing gesture, perhaps wrinkling the dress up a bit —*anything* to make you look like you're at ease with what you're wearing.

A good model knows how to make a photograph come alive. She can't just stand there like a doll or a wax effigy, one hand on her hip and the other on her hair. Successful models, even if they're stiffly posed with accessories and pins and wires holding everything in place, have and use an innate sense of timing. They have a rapport, or at least a communication, with the photographer, and know instinctively when he's going to take the picture. Every photographer has his own particular rhythm. At the moment his shutter snaps, the model's whole body—hands, feet, smile, glance, and outfit—should fall into place.

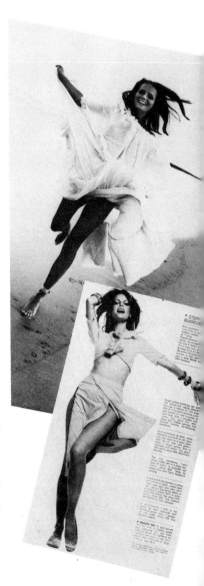

Modeling is for the most part an exciting and a broadening profession, but this doesn't mean there aren't going to be frustrations and disappointments— slow periods, delays, postponements. You may have to invest money in photographic composites and transportation and hair salons and clothes before you earn anything to speak of. And you don't get to keep the clothes you model, which are valuable samples belonging to the designer. You will be rejected not once but often, and you will have to learn not to take this too personally. Once you are established, your career will demand grueling work and self-discipline. If you regularly stay out till dawn, dissipation will in- evitably register in your face. I've always loved staying out late, but I often had to sacrifice my social life to my early-morning bookings. A model's working day is long and arduous. Few people outside the profession realize the pressures, the numbers of collaborators with different ideas, the patience it takes to stand in position while hairdressers, stylists, editors, makeup artists, clients, and photographers fuss and fiddle with you.

Frequently a shooting session lasts eight hours, and can stretch to ten. There have been moments when I didn't think I could stand one more brushing by the hairdresser. You'll need stamina and, above all, *pa- tience* to survive as a model. And a good business sense, too. Having a pretty face is only part of the job.

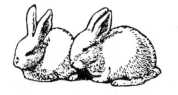

# 2

## Getting It Together

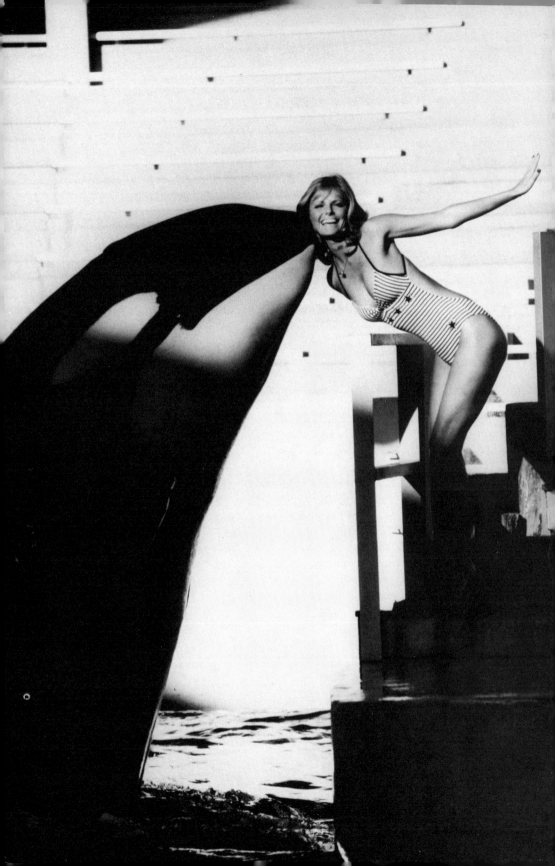

Appearances are not all-important, but they are definitely important. The first thing we perceive about other people is how they look. Psychologists have done studies that indicate that in general people find physically attractive men and women kinder, stronger, more intelligent and more outgoing than others. And there can be no denying that good-looking people have an easier time of it getting jobs and making social contacts. If they happen to be smart and have a pleasing personality as well, then the world is not only an open door for them, it's their "oyster, their champagne, their caviar."

We're all of us more confident about ourselves when we know we're looking good. Others in turn are persuaded by our fine display of self-esteem (one reason it works like a charm is that we have very often first had to persuade *ourselves!*). The more we get out of ourselves, the better able we are to relate to others. But sadly, there are those who do not feel as attractive as they actually are, and others who don't take the time and make the effort necessary to look their best.

I believe that just about anyone can be attractive. There are no absolute standards of beauty. Women who seem beautiful to us have often simply learned the art of making themselves alluring. They have learned to express the positive aspects of their personalities in the way they dress, wear their hair and makeup, and carry themselves. They have the glamour of their own identity.

Growing up, I often had those old chestnuts "Beauty is only skin deep" and "Pretty is as pretty does" flung willy-nilly at me. But when I stopped dodging them and actually thought about them, I realized they were true. And certainly, the way a woman looks is not the *most* important thing about her. God knows, great beauties can be calculating, manipulative, dissembling, or just plain dishwater-dull; and when they are, their beauty is diminished, the gilt peels off the statue (going, going, gone!). A less-than-perfect nose, slightly crooked teeth, a higher-than-high forehead, when they are those of someone we love, can be beautiful to us. We no longer look at them critically, for the spell of love is everywhere.

Physical beauty can be something of a double-edged sword. It is often the mother of complacency and the

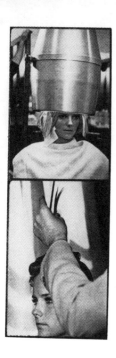

sire of lack-of-development: enter the living doll who just sits around attracting jocks like flies while her tongue melts and her brain atrophies. Sure she has an edge over the rest of the field, but there are dangers lying in wait for her—half-hidden, implicit, often unrecognized until too late. Don't get me wrong, I'm all for good looks but not when they're used as a shield or crutch or short-term weapon.

The landscape of a woman's face is composed of many things—her smile, the light in her eyes, the way she holds her head: in a word, her *character*. That makes every woman responsible for her own face. Classic features, a great figure, and even youth, with the grace *it* confers, can all spell emptiness. Soon enough we'll all be old—wrinkles will inevitably develop and muscle tone go—and unless there is an ever-developing brain, what will we have left?

A couple of years ago, *Harper's Bazaar* came out with a list of the "Ten Most Beautiful Women." They were: Lauren Hutton, Elizabeth Taylor, Faye Dunaway, Diahann Carroll, Candice Bergen, Princess Grace of Monaco, Ali MacGraw, Cheryl Tiegs, Lena Horne, and Farrah Fawcett. I was very gratified to be included because the women were all individuals who had built on what they had in order to make the most of themselves and their lives; it wasn't the symmetry of their faces and bodies that made them beautiful and alive—it was what was going on inside them.

Some women have just the knack for creating a style that expresses their nature in a very *contemporary* way. Others have unconsciously formed habits and attitudes and fixed patterns of living and looking that all but bury them alive. Often the mistakes they make—again and again, in many cases—are ones that some honest self-analysis could help win a victory over.

## MISTAKES PEOPLE MAKE

### Overfocusing on Flaws

Don't become obsessed with a feature or a part of your body you dislike. A beautiful model I know used to go around claiming she had a "droopy eye," that it was · ruining the symmetry of her face. No matter how hard I looked, I could never discover which eye it was she was talking about.

Try transferring your gaze and attention to whatever *assets* you possess in the most natural setting on earth—your own person.

## Projecting an "Uncomfortable" Look

Any look that requires a lot of extra effort to carry off —be it in the hair, eye shadow, lipstick, or wardrobe department—is ultimately going to catch you out. Every woman has found herself in this predicament; the moment comes when she can't imagine what she could have been imagining when she got herself together in the first place. Recently, because they were in style, I went and bought some "gathered" skirts, the kind I've always disliked. When I actually put one of them on, I felt completely lost in it—and it served me right. Once, I said okay when a hairdresser asked to tease and spray my hair before a party; he promised I would never regret it, never look back. I looked like a spider's web, a sparrow's nest, a pumpkinhead—all that hair just wasn't me, I couldn't relax and be myself. Following fads takes a toll, and you can't always be sure of applause, either.

There's a big difference, though, between forcing yourself to accommodate to a look and adapting to a positive change of style in hair, makeup, or wardrobe.

Changes, even when you know you need them, may make you feel uncomfortable right off. Only time will tell you whether you just need to adjust to your new look, or whether you really did make a mistake. We're all entitled to a few mistakes. The thing is not to make a fine art out of making them.

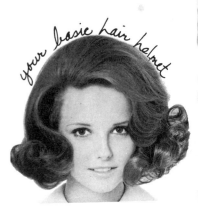

your basic hair helmet

## Resisting Change

Yes, you always run the risk of bungling the job when you attempt to change your basic look, but the biggest mistake, in my opinion, is not changing your look at all, ever. Your appearance should reflect both the changes for the better going on inside you and the changes in taste in the world at large. Few of us feel the same way we felt a decade ago—so why should we stand still and be a walking advertisement for interchangeability? Taste has many provinces, and some of them are difficult to reconcile: how, for instance, can you keep abreast of current styles and also preserve your individual taste? The first step is not to typecast yourself unfairly by modeling yourself on a figure from the past, even your own past. I'm not telling you to rush out and in a confused moment acquire every cosmetic and accessory mentioned in the latest fashion magazine you happen to have read. On the other hand, you really do want to try to avoid looking like a dinosaur.

## Neglecting the Basics of Good Health

Extra fat usually goes hand in hand with less than perfect skin, unhealthy color, dreary hair and a crying lack of mobility and animation. These are the signs—and there are no mistaking them—of poor nutrition and lack of exercise: ignore them at your peril. Only in a fairy tale does fat disappear by itself. In real life, it glaringly points out that you have somewhere along the line lost your belief in your own attractiveness.

Overweight and other problems caused by bad nutrition and lack of exercise are less "mistakes" than they are the result of a sometimes criminal neglect, lack of discipline, and lack of knowledge about health practices. What extra pounds say to me (and I know—remember, I carried more than my share of them around with me for a couple of years) is, "I don't care enough! I don't know enough!" And it follows that if *you* neglect the way you look, you're extending an invitation to others to neglect you, too. It might help to bear in mind that the biggest essential of natural beauty is good health.

## Not Spending Enough on Your Appearance

Enough what? Not money. Time and attention. Throughout this book I'll be suggesting different ways for you to approach the problem of your appearance: by studying and analyzing yourself, by experimenting, and finally, by getting professional advice when necessary. But nothing I say is going to make a whit of difference unless you program yourself to spend the time it takes to work on the ideas I throw out. But once you decide to invest the time to work out the general look that's most becoming to you, putting yourself together on a day-to-day basis should take only a few minutes. My point is, you can't just close your eyes and open them again and find yourself transformed.

Spending a lot of money to look your best is not necessary. We all know women who manage to put themselves together brilliantly on a shoestring (and some divine inspiration), and we also know their opposites, women who have obviously spent hard, cold cash—and lots of it—to make themselves alluring, and who have failed ignominiously. Conspicuous consumption is out these days; what's in is taking the measure of what's available and using it to make the most of what you have to offer.

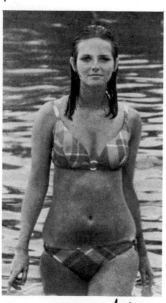

"*before*"

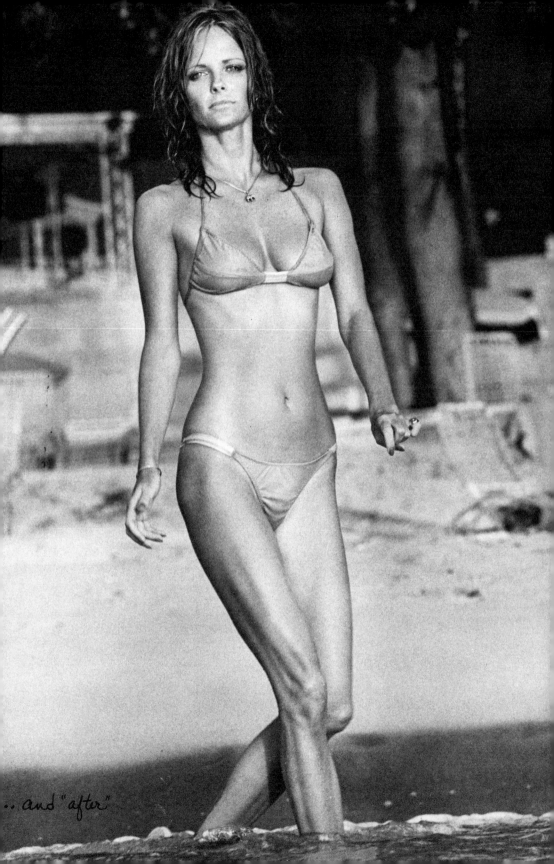

*.. and "after"*

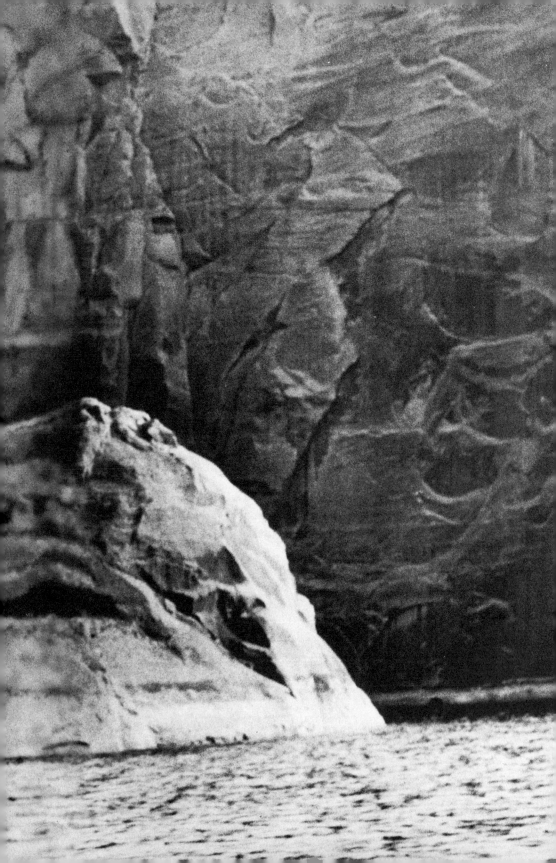

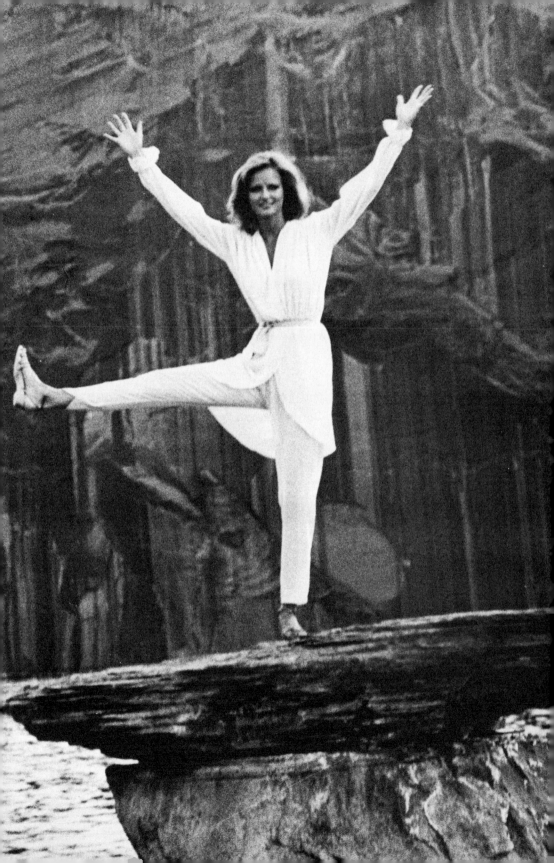

Women sometimes change their look at random, without adequate thought or preparation—sometimes out of reaction to a bad day or a low mood; the change itself will generally repay the compliment by making them look not better but worse. So don't let yourself be a sandwich board for your inner confusions and private disasters.

Instead, imagine yourself in the most positive terms. Coming up with a look to express your personality is going to be a bit tricky if you have never fully understood yourself or if you tend to think of yourself in terms of your faults, failings, and faux pas. When you think of yourself, don't think "No! No! No!" but rather, "Yes! Yes! Yes!" I used to think of myself as a shy person, and "shy" to me had a negative, thwarted connotation. Now I think of it as meaning cautious, not pushy, etc. If I'd attuned myself to hear only the negative implications of "shy," I might be wearing drab clothes and dull makeup today, all the better to recede into the woodwork. As it is, I prefer somewhat conservative styles, muted colors, and soft, understated fabrics, but I know full well the value of an occasional splash of color and of wearing what I call "energy clothes."

So: don't run yourself down and don't drag yourself down to where you can't get up and walk on. Consider how you would represent yourself on a job interview. Would you describe yourself as aggressive? Aren't dynamic and vivacious more positive terms, connoting the sort of attitude an employer would want you to bring to the job? And wouldn't you describe yourself as calm and relaxed instead of introverted? If you think of yourself as uncreative, ask why you're so confident of your own uncreativity. And maybe you're zany instead of scatterbrained, thoughtful instead of aloof, honest and direct instead of tactless and brash. Describe yourself as you would describe someone you loved and you may just find out that you *are* describing someone you love: yourself.

Now ask yourself which of your physical characteristics you're happiest with. Do you have eyes that are a nice color? A slender waist? Long legs? A clear skin with smooth coloration? Full lips? A beautiful bosom? Lustrous long hair? Whatever . . .

Dwell on the parts of yourself that you may have been ignoring and work back from there. Forget about the flaws—for *now*. There are bound to be things you don't like about yourself—try to redefine them in positive terms. Place them at your service: try to see yourself as voluptuous instead of fat (remember Rubens!), petite instead of too small, slender instead of skinny. Find flattering adjectives to describe your face, and then your body. Now is the time to be generous to yourself—so you'll be in a better position psychologically later on to deal with the parts of yourself that even a switch in adjectives can't make you like.

## Believing That Beauty Is Unattainable

Don't rule out something because you've convinced yourself you can't achieve it. Don't allow some mythical distance to be built up between you and a far-off end product. A human being is by definition a "living contradiction of rules and prejudices, and everything that is human is a special case." I urge you to consider that beauty and glamour are like almost everything else in that they require a step-by-step process that is *not*—I repeat *not*—beyond your reach. Don't feel bound by what *you've* decided are your limitations. Most of those glamorous magazine cover girls came from Kansas and Kalamazoo; they struggled from the word "go," and absorbed—through hard work and concentration—the details of the beauty industry. My advice is to follow up your dreams to the point where they become reality. It was Lillian Hellman, I think, who said the things in this world belong to the people who want them the most.

Once you've focused on your good points and are beginning to feel like someone who can set out to do something and then actually get it done, begin scrutinizing the women you know whose looks and clothes you admire, as well as fashion models, actresses, and strangers you see on the street or at parties. What is it about them that traps your attention, pleases your eye, and in rare cases even lays claim to your imagination? Is it the way they wear their makeup, clothes, or hair, or something more elusive—the way they speak, the gestures they use? And above all, notice how what they wear complements their personality. Do they strike you as being able to live up to their trimmings?

One difficulty is that most people have preconceived notions of how they look and have little or no idea how others see them. Many of us simply think of ourselves the way our parents and friends have "seen" us all our lives. If we were made to feel awkward and unattractive during our formative years, we may go on feeling awkward and unattractive, however unblemished the rest of our lives has been. Some of us continue to see ourselves in terms of a beauty problem that afflicted us long ago. For example, long after I lost all those extra pounds, I saw myself as overweight. And I think that many other women look in the mirror and see a self that no longer exists except insofar as it prevents them from seeing their real and better selves. To compound matters, since they can't see themselves as they are, they can't make the right changes—or even discern good advice when they hear it, as I've noticed from when giving out beauty tips every Thursday morning on *Good Morning America*. I might say something like, "If you have a round face, don't wear a round hat." And the next day someone with a round face will come up to me and tell me how much they enjoyed the day before's program—*wearing a round hat!* They just don't see themselves realistically enough to realize that the recommendation applied to *them*.

But how can you possibly see yourself as others see you? One way is to use your acting potential and glance into the mirror (the best critic there is, the only truly honest friend) and pretend that you're a stranger to yourself. Then act out various scenarios in front of the mirror: imagine you're walking into a room, or sitting down, or talking to someone you've just met by chance, or looking at a painting in a museum, or waiting for a bus. Smile, grimace, laugh, frown—how do you look? Run the gamut from clown to tragedian. The old mirror won't betray you, and your perception of yourself may become more realistic.

Now you can stop play-acting, theater-time's up. You're you again, your one-true-first-last-only self. Move closer to the mirror and examine yourself for areas that you *know* could use improvement. A close look at your body may reveal the beginnings of problems that just aren't visible when you have layers of clothes on. Chances are those specters will indicate that you could use a good diet, some more exercise, and some good old "R and R." Now look very closely at your face. It should be clean and without makeup. Don't get depressed—we all need work, and not everything in life is as pleasant as licking ice cream.

Studying a photograph of yourself is yet another way of learning something about the visual impression you make on others. You may see you have your mouth open or a false smile, a mannerism of one kind or another you never realized was yours. "Surprise" photographs are the most useful—the ones that have been taken without your having had time to "pose." Are your shoulders slumped down? Are you sitting up straight? Is your belt halfway up to your neck? Is your stomach sticking out? A photo that has caught you animatedly talking to someone may reveal in capsule form the way you look to others.

Also, criticism—although you may not always delight in it—when you are trying to work out a look for yourself, is indispensable and should be taken seriously. I'm talking about constructive criticism from your friends, something as far from idle flattery as it is from insult and injury. Photographers, stylists, fellow models, makeup artists, hairdressers, and other professionals in the fashion world have given me great ideas. And my husband also happens to have a good sense of fashion and has always been quick to point out if I had anything on that would take away from my kind of casualness. Close friends have an eerie way of knowing if you really want to know what they think or are just fishing for compliments. Cosmeticians and salesgirls often have good ideas but since they don't know you, they may recommend some weirdo fashion slant that will start you on the road to becoming a great big phony.

Keep an open mind. Embrace the suggestions that seem right to you and discard those that you don't feel comfortable with. In order to please others, you have to please yourself. And pleasing yourself entails knowing exactly who and what you are. Then and only then will you be ready to act on this understanding.

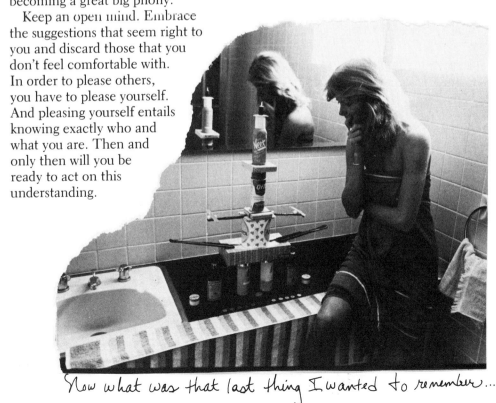

Now what was that last thing I wanted to remember...

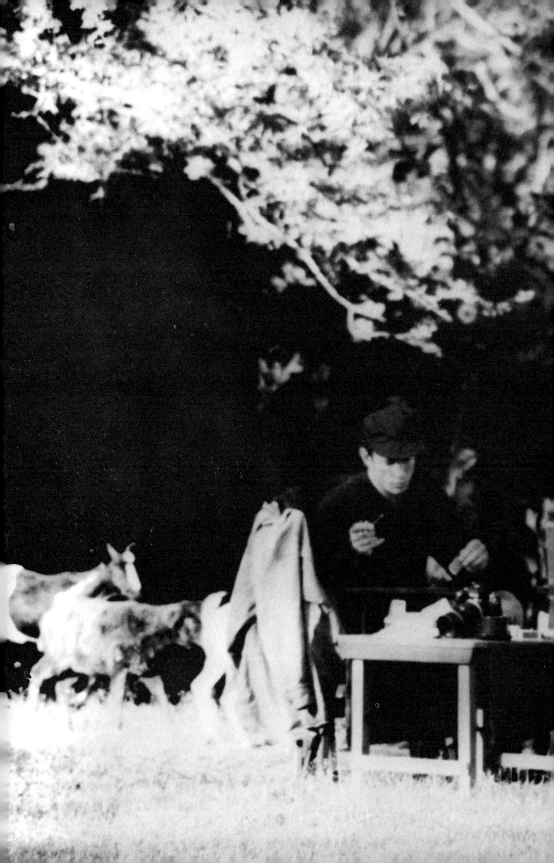

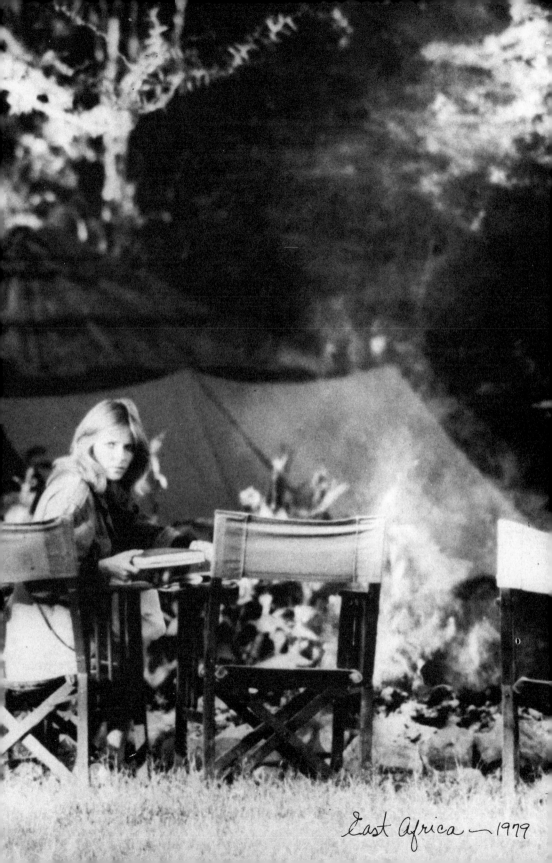

East africa — 1979

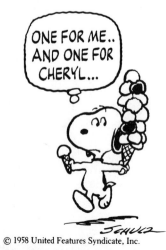

3

# Food Therapy and Eating Strategy: Advice to the Food-lorn

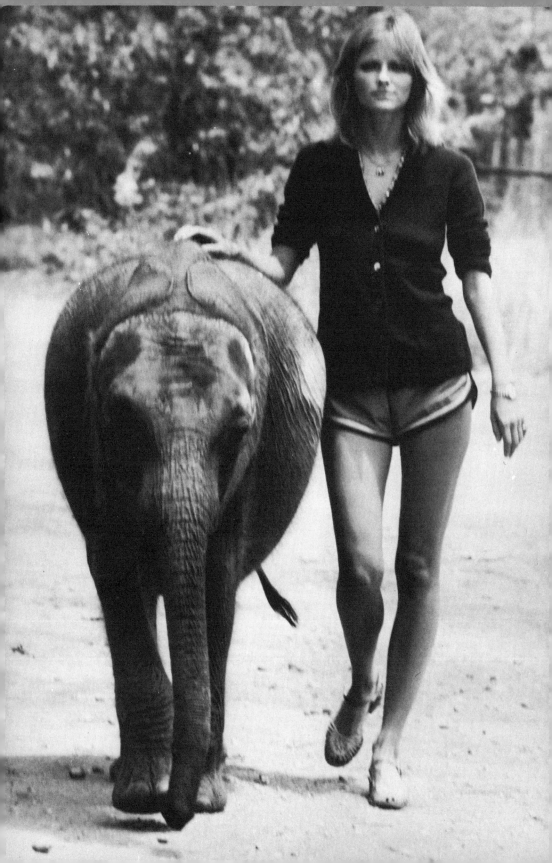

_s_ there a woman alive who would rather be fat than thin? I doubt it. A body without extra padding is the most pleasing to look at; it also gives off an aura of health and dynamic vitality that makes people want to be around you. A slender form may be a thing of beauty but it doesn't happen all by itself; rather, it is the result of exercise and a low-calorie diet.

A good diet, however, is not just one that keeps you thin, but one that is also nutritious and provides you with the energy that today's super-active women need. Many women suffer (_and need not suffer_) not only from overweight but from its grim accompaniments as well: frayed nerves, assorted digestive problems, poor skin, weak nails, lifeless hair, and so on. Diet-related health and beauty problems are often caused by lack of knowledge as to just what food _does_ in your body. But it doesn't have to be this way.

## HOW MUCH DO YOU KNOW ABOUT YOUR DIET?

■ _Allow 100 pounds for the first five feet of your height. Add three pounds for each additional inch. This is your ideal weight. Now: How far do you exceed it?_

■ _Does your weight vacillate by ten or more pounds several times in the course of a year?_

■ _Do you shed a lot of weight in a short, concentrated period of time with some "miracle diet"—only to regain it?_

■ _Do you know how many calories there are in a hamburger on a roll? In an average serving of fish? In an apple? In a doughnut? In a cup of sweetened breakfast cereal?_

■ _Do you know approximately how many calories there are in the total amount of food you consume (including liquids) in an average day?_

■ _Do you know which foods contain Vitamin A? Fiber? All the B vitamins? Calcium?_

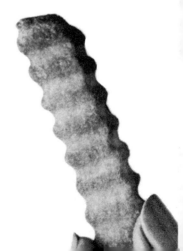

■ *Do you suffer frequently from heartburn? Constipation? Headaches?*

■ *Are you often irritable? Depressed? Lethargic?*

■ *Are you apt to overeat when you're feeling lonely or bored?*

I have a lot of suggestions on how to turn around your behavior patterns. First of all, if your weight is not "ideal" and you were unable to give the total calorie count of the food you eat, you've probably already discovered one very big reason why you're overweight: You are eating a lot more calories than you think you are.

If you are slender and feel great you must be doing something right, or else your lack of knowledge hasn't caught up with you—yet. This chapter should provide you with some of what you need to know in order to *stay* thin and healthy. A new awareness of the food you eat can only improve the way you look and feel. The rest of the package is motivation, discipline, and sheer old-fashioned guts.

## MY VERY OWN BATTLE OF THE BULGE

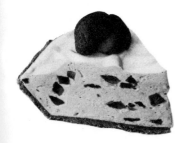

When I was overweight I would have flunked the preceding questionnaire gloriously. I ate whatever and whenever I wanted to, and as not too much else was going on in my lazy life, most of what I did was eat. But my worst sins lay in not knowing about nutrition and in never considering how what I was and wasn't eating would make me feel.

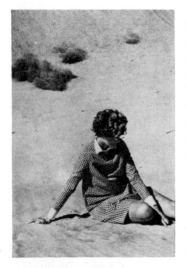

My binge-eating syndrome came into its own in college. I started each day with a huge, satisfying breakfast—the only problem was it didn't even begin to satisfy me. Between every morning class I would pay a little visit to the handy candy machine. I could hardly wait till lunchtime. First, I would demolish whatever I'd brought from home, then I'd repair to the snack bar for some hot-buttered popcorn or ice cream—I needed that extra incentive to go back to class with its routine of note-taking and lecture-listening. The good thing about candy bars was they could easily be transported from English Lit. to Psychology 1A and so on. I was still pretty skinny—I guess I was burning up most of the calories with the flame of youthful energy or something—and I never gave a thought to how much I was consuming.

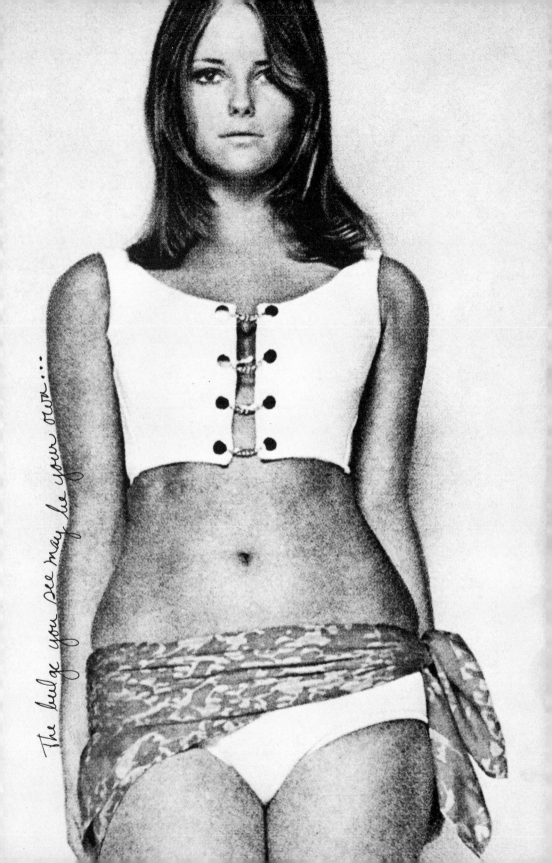

The bulge you see may be your own...

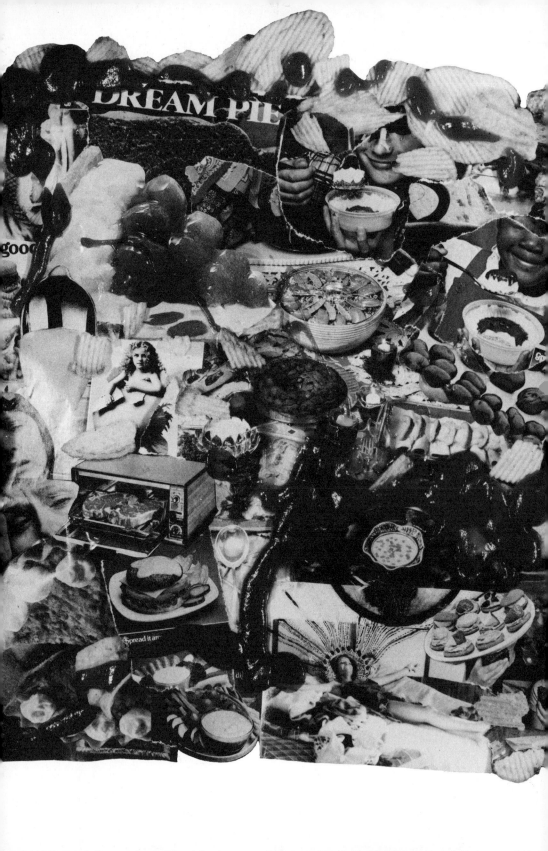

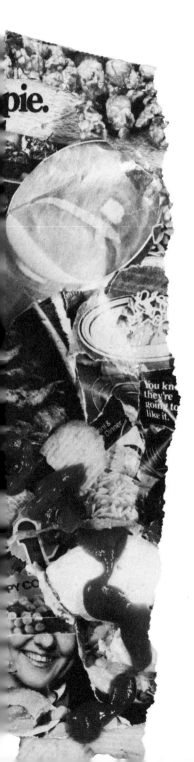

When I went to live and model in New York at the age of nineteen, however, the tons of junk I was forever eating began to catch up with me. My body had reached its full growth and now I could no longer burn off the inordinate number of calories I was shoveling in. The extra pounds that had congregated around my midriff and thighs didn't stop me—I naïvely thought it must be my metabolism. And as for any anxiety I felt, I simply fed it—literally as well as figuratively!

Thinking back on these tales of the Burger Princess, I'm amazed at the amount of food I managed to choke down. I loved veal parmesan, breaded, with lots of cheese and sauce. And I loved noshing on combination pizzas and double-decker Big Macs with ketchup and mayonnaise. I never thought about the difference in calories between steak and fish, between potatoes and broccoli (with plenty of hollandaise, naturally—I mean, *unnaturally!*), or between tomato and orange juice: to me it was all the same—it was, in a word, *food!* I loved banana splits, butterscotch sundaes, hot-fudge sundaes with whipped cream, nuts, and, topping it all off, the maraschino cherry, which sometimes I ate and sometimes I didn't (I'd already concluded that almost anything anyone does with a maraschino cherry is symbolic). I loved doughnuts and I ordered them pumped full of whipped cream and dipped in deep, dark chocolate. But most of all I loved cherry pie à la mode. I wasn't fussy, though. When they didn't have my favorites on hand, I'd order at random and in bulk and often quite wildly—cookies with peanut butter, Ritz Crackers with Hellmann's Mayonnaise and bread-and-butter pickles. As long as there was a *lot* of it, I loved it. I remember visiting a friend for the weekend and asking for double helpings of every single course at both lunch and dinner. *"Cheryl,"* my friend said, leaving it at that. Later that night, I felt the old urge and sneaked downstairs in the deep dark of the unfamiliar house, longing for the feel of the icebox door, the pulling of the handle and the clicking on of the inside light—it would be like coming home. The range of possibilities was disappointingly limited: jars of mustard, pots of margarine, vegetable trays of zucchini and rhubarb—nothing that could be immediately eaten. If only there had been a potato, I could have peeled and devoured it with salt. Way in the back was an old box of after-dinner mints. They must have been in there for about a year because the chocolate was starting to turn moldy. I ate one and

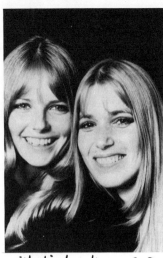

with Liz Landis — 1968

then another and another of the tasteless sweets until I saw that more than half the wrappers were empty; I nervously arranged them so they'd look as much as possible like the same old mess I'd happened upon. Then, I quietly shut the fridge and in total darkness crept upstairs to bed, thinking of course of the remaining sweets which I had a feeling I would meet again.

After I was married, I continued to overeat. I was a bad influence on my slim husband and he gained, too. We'd spend weekends lounging around our apartment ordering in sundaes, pastries, pizzas. I guess you could have called ours "The Catered Affair." Or else "Getting Fat Together."

By now I had begun to worry about the extra pounds, but worrying only made me hungry, even while I was gorging. Unlike most binge eaters, I had an economic reason to fear those pounds. They were threatening to blight my budding career. In retrospect, I think that I ate to try to fill up an empty space —not in my stomach but in my soul, because whenever I felt anxious, depressed, or insecure, I ate: speed eating—food on the run, food on the fly (toy food on planes), and, going overboard, bulk food on ships.

One Christmas I went home to visit my family in California. My older sister, Vernette, had always been a bit heavier than I, but that year, when she giddily tried on my skirts, they were swimming on her. With my heart in my mouth, I went into the bathroom and stepped on the scale for the first time in months (binge eaters for obvious reasons don't like to weigh themselves) and, my God, I saw the needle hover at and come to rest on the 150 mark. I burst into tears! Then, not unnaturally, I marched into the kitchen and ate everything in sight, including an entire box of See's candy. It was like I was officiating at my own funeral.

Sometimes I actually scare myself by recalling things like how on a trip to Puerto Rico for a bathing suit issue I raided the cupboards of a house we had rented in the old section of the island; no one human had been living there for a while and insects were hatching inside the boxes of crackers on the shelf. And what did I do? I ate around them! Ugh!!

My roommate of those days in New York, Liz Landis, can vouch for my abilities as a disposal unit. Somebody once sent her a box of cookies from Paris and she ate out their gooey insides and threw the crusts into the garbage can. When I got home that night, I caught a glimpse of these castaways and one by one extracted them from the garbage and finished them off. Some had the flavor of orange peels, others of coffee grind, but soon they were gone, and I remember standing there afterwards feeling thoroughly ashamed of myself—as if I'd just committed some form of gustatory rape.

During this time, I was afflicted by migraine headaches. I spent a lot of time in agony in bed, and was constantly having to refill prescriptions for painkillers. I had the idea that hearty eating would make the violent headaches disappear; so, whenever I felt one coming on, I'd order up a hamburger smothered in onions.

Then my mother confided that every time she ate ice cream she got a headache. I looked at her and thought, maybe that's it—or part of it, anyway. I've since realized that my body simply couldn't handle all the sugar I'd sent flooding through it. When I changed my eating habits, my migraines all but vanished. Now, when I feel a headache coming on, I stop eating altogether, take a single aspirin, and nip it in the bud.

My binging habits also blemished my skin and made me feel tired. My remedy for lethargy was my old familiar one—a candy bar or a sundae.

So now you know how I know what it feels like to be a foodaholic. But don't despair, there is light at the end of the tunnel—your days as an obsessive muncher in public and a compulsive muncher in private can definitely be put behind you (instead of on your behind).

When I first tried to diet, I failed, because my diet was based on as little knowledge of nutrition as my abnormal eating habits had been. For breakfast I would have "only" a corn muffin (plastered with butter and jelly) and I would take care to eat "only" one or two desserts a day. When this "diet" didn't produce results, I devised others. Sometimes I just skipped breakfast altogether and went as long as I could without eating anything at all. But total abstinence made me feel tired and irritable, and, needless to say, very, very hungry, so that when I finally did eat, I ate as though I was starving, which in fact I was. Once I tried a "no-meat diet," because some self-styled expert had told me that meat was fattening. So whenever I ordered Eggs Benedict—a super-rich concoction of English Muffins, ham, poached eggs, and hollandaise sauce, I virtuously stripped away the little piece of ham —content in the sure knowledge that it was this torn flesh of pig that was causing the trouble.

The next mistake I made was "diet-hopping." I went

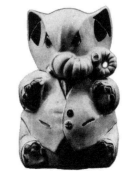

my elephant cookie jar.

out and bought every diet book on the market and read them all. (I used to joke that my real problem was always what to eat while reading the latest diet book.) Name a diet, and I've been on it: the grapefruit diet, the all-meat-and-water diet, the all-fat diet, the all-juice diet, the yogurt diet. But after a few days of rigorous self-denial, I'd be right back where I started—in the refrigerator, cleaning out the leftovers. By the law of averages, *some* of the diets I tried, such as the Weight Watcher's diet, were quite sensible, but I never lost weight on any of them because I supplemented them with the "Cheryl Tiegs Diet"—*lots* of junk food and multiple snacks. At one point I even went to a "diet doctor," who prescribed diet pills containing the dangerous stimulant, amphetamine. In this post-Doctor-Feelgood decade, most people know that the diet pill syndrome can be addictive, but in the sixties, few realized this. Most models took amphetamines, not to mention Vitamin B-12 shots. My mistake was thinking that since I was taking diet pills, I didn't have to diet. So I continued eating as before. I lost a bit of weight, yes—but not nearly enough. It was ludicrous. The doctor could see that the boxes of multi-colored amphetamines he'd prescribed for me had all been consumed, and he must have been wondering why my face and body were still blubbery.

Finally I reached the point of total desperation. None of the diets I'd attempted on my own had worked; if anything, I was getting fatter. I would contemplate my hips and thighs and chins and just cry. I felt really terrible about myself. I resolved to take the matter (meaning me) in hand, and I enrolled in a diet clinic in New York—determined to eat *only* what the doctor told me I could.

The clinic weighed me in every day and gave me a shot of special vitamins and nutrients (no amphetamine). Every noon I received a bag of food, containing my lunch and dinner—a total of 400 nutritious calories. Lunch was a small piece of fish or meat, a tiny whole-wheat cracker, and a little side dish of vegetables. Ditto dinner, with two pieces of fruit thrown in. I stuck to that diet for an entire month. Nothing —and I *mean* nothing—that wasn't in my bag passed my lips. When I went to parties, I didn't drink a thing, and when I went to restaurants I carted along my little bag. At the end of just one month I'd lost twenty pounds. After that I gradually increased my intake of calories. I won't easily forget how terrified I was that I'd gain weight again, when I sipped my first glass of

I HAVE A NEW DIET...YOU CAN EAT ANYTHING YOU WANT, BUT YOU CAN'T SWALLOW!

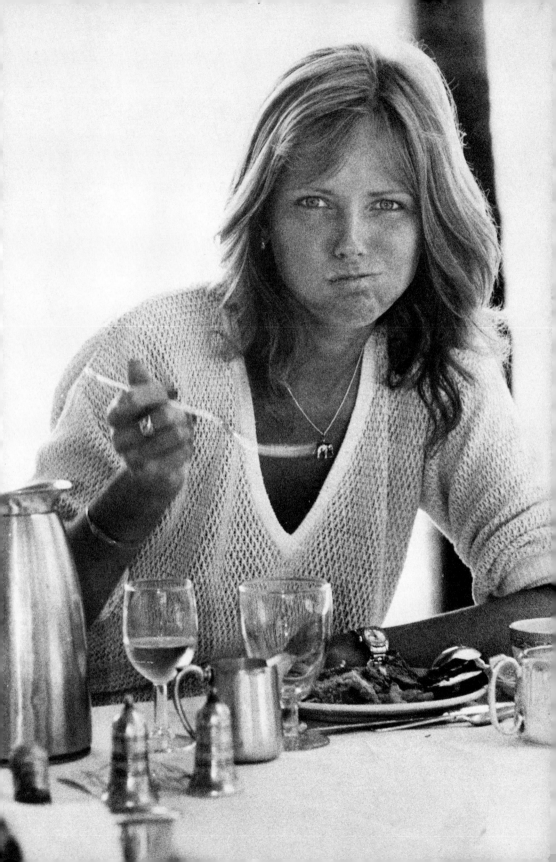

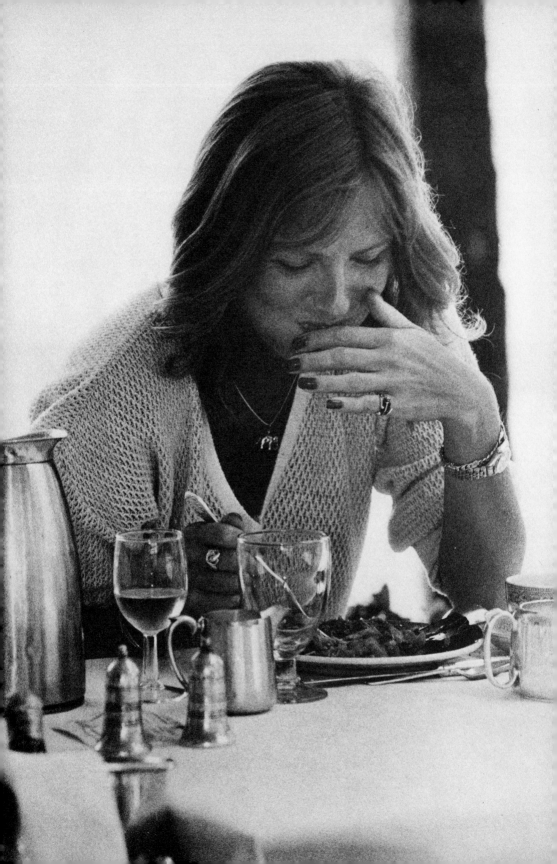

wine and tasted my first morsel that didn't come from my clinical feedbag. But I never did regain that weight. I was so happy to be thin again I never returned to binging. The pattern was broken, the neurotic cycle destroyed.

I don't think it's necessary for everyone to enroll in a diet clinic in order to lose weight. I now see that it was my determination to become thin again, my sheer need to overcome, that made me stop overeating. Without that desperate need, the clinic's diet would have been as useless to me as all the other diets I'd tried. I think I might even have lost those first twenty pounds a little too quickly for my own good. Nutritionists consider it safest for dieters to lose weight slowly, two pounds a week at most, over a long period of time, to avoid the risk of depleting nutritional reserves. Fortunately, the shots the clinic gave me preserved the delicate balance of vitamins and nutrients in my system. Also, I was young. I suffered no ill effects from this sudden weight loss—such as sagging skin and dry, brittle hair.

What was invaluable about the clinic is that it taught me the type and amount of food that was both nutritious and low in calories. I have continued with my study of nutrition, and find the subject endlessly fascinating. I am far too aware of what the quantities of junk food I'd been eating had done to me—physiologically and psychologically—to ever eat that way again. I consider myself one of the lucky ones.

## THE MATHEMATICS OF A GOOD DIET

Arithmetic has never been my forte, but I've discovered that maintaining a slender figure requires some simple math. Calculate the number of pounds you should weigh and the number of calories you should eat to stay thin.

As I suggested in the questionnaire, ideal body weight can be roughly computed by allowing 100 pounds for the first five feet of height and three pounds for each additional inch. Since I am 5'10", my ideal weight is 130. When you've computed your ideal weight you'll notice that it's considerably less than the weight advocated by the charts in your doctor's office. You should know that those weights are based on insurance company charts, and they tend to be high, insomuch as they reflect the fact that the average American (25,000,000 of him!) is overweight. Of

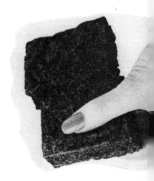

course, if you are large-boned and have very broad shoulders, a large pelvic structure, and big ankles and wrists, you may look better when you do weigh a bit more. But since I am relatively small-boned and spend a lot of my working day in front of a camera, which automatically puts about ten extra pounds on you, I feel more comfortable at 120 pounds. So adjust these "ideal" figures to suit your body build, but don't leave room for fat—we all know a bulge when we see one.

A good diet also calls for some addition and subtraction. Let's imagine you need to lose ten pounds to reach your ideal weight. According to nutritionists, a pound of stored fat contains 3500 calories. For every pound you want to lose, then, you must cut back your present calorie consumption by 3500 calories over a period of time. Only when those calories have *not* been taken in will you drop the pound. For example, if you take in 2000 calories a day and cut them back to 1500 calories a day, you will have eliminated 3500 calories, or shed one pound, in seven days. At this rate it will take you ten weeks to lose ten pounds. You will have cut a total of 35,000 calories out of your diet in two and a half months. You must also get into the habit of counting the calories you eat and estimating the calories you use up. Though we tend to think of a calorie as a little fat-producing demon, what it actually is is a positive unit of energy. Calories supply the fuel our bodies need to move, work, think, and otherwise function; we can't live without them. Calories that are not put to work and burned off, however, do get retained as fat. Different types of calories, such as those in starches and sugar, are more likely to turn to fat than are others; and naturally, different types of activities burn calories at different rates.

In general, sedentary activities (sitting, writing, watching TV, reading) burn about 60 calories per hour; light housework (dusting, sewing, ironing) and walking at a normal pace burn about 160 calories per hour. Moderate activities (walking briskly, golfing, shopping, calisthenics, biking at a slow pace) and heavier housework (sweeping, making beds) burn from 280 to 350 calories per hour. More vigorous activities and sports (disco dancing, fast biking, energetic tennis, chopping wood) burn about 450 calories per hour. The real calorie burners and the ones that aid and abet your dieting are squash, paddleball, swimming (a fast crawl), and serious jogging, all of which burn 600

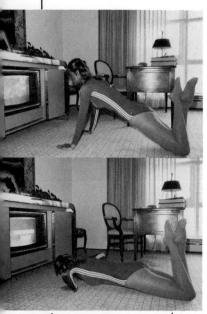

Don't just sit there — do something.

or more calories per hour. You also burn calories while you sleep, but very few—about 30 per hour.

Therefore, if you sit at a desk eight hours a day, walk home from work, clean the house, cook the dinner, and then collapse in front of the TV, your total calorie expenditure for the day is low. If, on top of this, you nibble Danish pastries at your desk, stop for a hot dog on your way home, munch a bunch of peanuts before dinner, and eat three meals a day, you don't have to be an Einstein to figure out that you will probably be gaining rather than losing weight. A bit of work with a pocket calculator will soon tell you whether or not you're consuming more fuel than you can burn up.

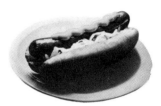

To complicate matters, when your body reaches maximum growth it will burn fewer calories, many calories having been burned up by the growing process itself. Moreover, when you are young, you tend to be active—running, jumping, playing all the time. As you get older and become more sedentary, more set—and seated—in your ways, you need fewer calories to maintain your body weight. Some experts maintain that to keep the slender figure you had at age eighteen, you must eat a third less calories than you did then. Yet most people, as I did, continue to eat as much as they did when they were teenagers—or even more. Some people are blessed with a rapid basal metabolism, which means that their bodies burn calories rapidly, but these are few and far between—exceptions to the rule. Many of the overweight just don't realize that the body naturally needs less fuel as it gets older, and try to blame their extra pounds on their metabolism, an old scapegoat. When I first started gaining weight, I took all sorts of diagnostic tests in an effort to find out what on earth had gone haywire with my metabolism—a waste of money and time! The overwhelming odds are that if you're too fat you're simply consuming more calories than you need for fuel.

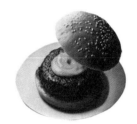

**73**

A low-calorie diet will allow most people to shed extra pounds. A 1200-calorie-a-day diet is considered a safe and effective reducing plan. Designing a palatable, energy-building 1200 calorie diet, however, requires some mathematical planning as well as some knowledge of food preparation. Not all calories are the same, and to stay healthy and look and feel your best, you must make sure you're burning high-quality fuel, packed with vitamins, minerals, and the other important nutritional elements.

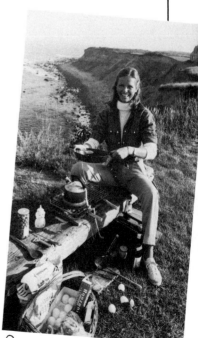

*From the frying pan...*

My first advice to dieters is to buy a pocket calorie counter. You may be suprised to learn how many calories foods you imagined were non-fattening contain. A half-pound club steak, for example, contains a walloping 670 calories! A piece of watermelon, which no one would ever dream could be fattening, is riddled with sugar and contains 100 calories per medium slice (and whoever heard of anyone's having a *medium* slice of watermelon?). Vegetables and lettuce, composed largely of water, are not a bit fattening, but the things that make them taste delicious—butter, mayonnaise, oil—are loaded with calories. Nuts, seeds, dates and granolas, which all health food fans celebrate, are positively (or negatively, as the case may be) bursting with calories. In general, there are four calories per gram in proteins and carbohydrates, and nine calories per gram in fats.

Many of the people who are struggling to lose weight already know the foods that are low in calories, but they do not know how much of it to eat. They know, for example, that cake, ice cream, pasta, and french fries are fatteners and therefore to be avoided, and that melon, veal, fish, and vegetables are on the whole slimming, health-giving foods. This is all perfectly true, but to diet successfully you must not only eliminate easily identified high-calorie treats but also measure and weigh low-calorie food. Most diets advise you to eat a quarter of a pound of meat, fish, or cheese with your main meals. A quarter of a pound is only *four tiny ounces*—a mini-mini-portion that no restaurant could ever get away with serving.

On the other hand, the caloric value of food is often disproportionate to its size. Sometimes the tiniest morsels are jam-packed with calories. A mere seven cashew nuts, for example, contain 75 calories (and show me the mortal who can stop at seven!). A strip of bacon contains 33 calories, two tablespoons of peanut butter 200, and a measly candy bar 260!

## COMPUTE YOUR WAY TO A SLIM FIGURE: GET READY, SET, GO!

If you really want to lose weight, I fervently recommend that you take the time and trouble to follow the formula below. A mathematical approach to dieting will not leave your extra pounds to luck or fate. With

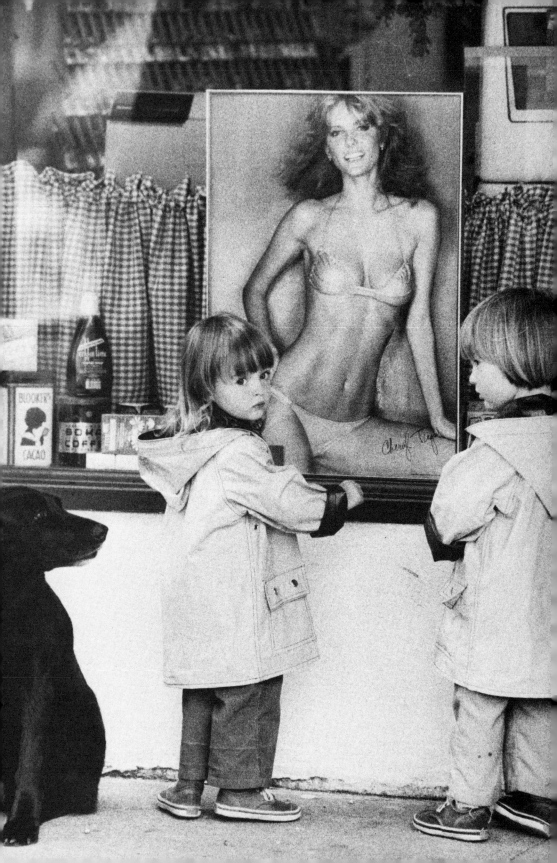

*this* system you will never be able to ignore the extra calories you consume, or the days you skip your exercises. And if you do not succeed in losing as much weight as you'd like, it will be easier to pinpoint the type of food you don't metabolize well and then to eliminate it from your diet.

Having computed your ideal weight according to formula, multiply the pounds you want to lose by 3500 calories. You now know the number of calories you must eliminate from your diet in order to lose your excess pounds.

Keep a record of what you eat for seven days; then, with your calorie counter, compute the number of calories you consumed. You are now in a position to figure out the approximate number of calories you burn in a single day. This is arguably more difficult, since metabolisms differ enormously, and there is a range for each bodily activity, depending on how quickly and vigorously you do it. If you are over twenty-five years old, I advise keeping your figures on the low side; even if they're not completely accurate, they'll give you a good idea of how many more calories you consume per day than you burn. If your food consumption and exercise quotient are likely to change drastically from day to day, compute a weekly average.

On the basis of the figures you now have, you should be able to decide just how many calories a day you can eat and still lose weight. The number of calories you eat per day should be lower than those you expend, but not lower than 1200 calories (the absolute minimum is 1000). Always remember that you must eliminate 3500 calories for each pound of fat you want to lose, and that the longer it takes you to eliminate those calories, the longer it's going to take to lose the unwanted weight. Don't plan on losing more than two pounds per week. A 1400–1500-calorie-a-day diet will enable you to lose weight, especially if you regularly consume more than that number of calories.

Plan a diet for yourself. Make a list of the low-calorie, nutritious foods that you *enjoy*, and of high-calorie junk fatteners that you know you must eliminate.

When you begin your diet, write down the caloric value of every kind of food—and that includes liquids, sauces, and dressings—that finds its way into your mouth. *Everything* you eat contains calories, except water, unsweetened coffee, and tea. You will of course need to know how *much* of a particular food you are eating. This isn't as complicated as it sounds. Note the weight of meat you buy and serve yourself a low-calorie portion. (Calorie counters contain helpful information.) Measure out dressings and fats with a tablespoon. Many breads, cereals, dairy products, and juices feature the caloric content per slice and eight-ounce cup right there on the package. Use a measuring cup. If necessary, buy a food scale.

When the great day comes and you find you've reached your ideal weight, compute the number of calories you can eat in order to maintain it: just multiply the desired number of pounds by twelve. If, for example, you want to stay at 123 pounds, you shouldn't eat more than 1476 (or 123 x 12) calories per day. (Now let's see, did anything historic happen in the year 1476?)

## THE LOW-CARBOHYDRATE DIET
---

Some people will not lose weight on a low-calorie diet if it includes such carbohydrates as bread, rice, pastas, potatoes, sugar, and alcohol. These people tend to retain salt in direct proportion to the amount of carbohydrates they consume, and when you retain salt, you retain water as well. And, as if that weren't enough, the body tends to convert carbohydrates to fat and store them.

If you need a low-carbohydrate diet (and you should let your doctor help you make this decision), lower your salt intake, and swear off sweets and refined starches, substituting unsaturated fats in the form of butterfat, beef, pork, and lamb. Don't make the mistake of eliminating *all* carbohydrates from your diet (they constitute a necessary and life-sustaining nutrient); just lower them to about two ounces a day—preferably complex carbohydrates, found in fruits, some vegetables, and whole grains.

## INVENT YOUR OWN!
---

You're the one who decides what you eat and when you eat it; what your food looks like and how it's seasoned. Every model I know has a scheme for maintaining her weight. Some prefer to skip breakfast and eat a large lunch. Others eat only one meal a day—dinner. Some eat six mini-meals a day. Others fast once a week. To each his own: Your patterns of food consumption *should* reflect your individual nature. If your diet doesn't feel right and also doesn't result in that slim figure you want, then it's obviously wrong for you. So change it.

A good, balanced diet should include a variety of foods. The real test of any diet is how it makes you feel. If you're tired, irritable, and go around the whole time with a "growling" stomach, you are clearly not taking in your fair share of essential nutrients. Ask yourself if you've taken the psychological factors into account. When you begin a diet you're bound to feel deprived, and your mind in turn is bound to communicate that feeling of deprivation to your stomach, making you "crave" the very foods that made you fat in the first place and that are tantalizingly out there waiting to make you fatter. Impatience and fatigue may very well beset you, but they are only temporary symptoms. Eventually your body will adjust to low-calorie food, and as soon as you start to lose weight in earnest, you'll feel happy with your new diet. When I long for a crunchy green salad, I obey my craving; but if it's a cookie I crave, I try to distract myself.

Whether or not you're trying to reduce, your body will tell you if you are eating the right foods. So do yourself a favor and listen to it. Many otherwise intelligent people fail to connect the way they feel with what they eat. The next time *you* feel run down, headachey, queasy, bloated or depressed, think back on the combinations of food you've eaten that day. In fact, don't wait until you're in extremity—check out your body after each meal. Note how sugar, proteins, fats, and heavy starches make you feel. A good diet will supply you with high-quality energy throughout the day.

## THE PERILS OF JUNK FOOD

Nutritionists define "junk" as food that contains an inordinate amount of refined sugar or refined grains, or food that has been stripped of its natural coating to make it last longer on the shelf. Unfortunately, the category of "junk food" encompasses most of the food-stuffs overweight people crave: ice cream, pancakes, spaghetti, white rolls, doughnuts, cake, candy, and on and on and on and on. These foods do absolutely nothing to build body tissue, add nothing to your bin of vitamins and nutrients, and convert easily to fat. Even worse, when you eat "junk" instead of nutritious food, you feel as hungry as you did before you indulged yourself. The reason for this is that refined sugars and

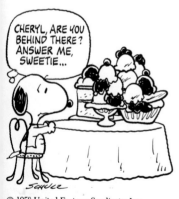

CHERYL, ARE YOU BEHIND THERE? ANSWER ME, SWEETIE...

starches are digested too rapidly and pour into the blood stream within minutes. Although the body's source of energy comes from sugar, or glucose, the body should be allowed to create glucose itself by slowly converting it from whole foods, and then to filter it gradually into the blood stream. But when you eat a candy bar to satisfy your hunger, the sugar hits your blood in a wave, the blood-sugar level rises rapidly, and you experience an increase of energy known in certain circles as a "high." The minute your pancreas registers this dramatic increase, it sends a flood of insulin, the hormone that controls the level of sugar in the blood, to manage the overdose. But because the pancreas has been overstimulated, it continues to send insulin after the job is done; and the insulin ends up obliterating *all* the sugar in your blood, with the result that you feel let-down, lethargic, and hungrier than ever. You reach for a food that will rapidly raise your blood sugar and restore your feeling of well-being— another candy bar! Is it any wonder that "junk food" is addictive? (Caffeine and alcohol have the same negative effect on blood sugar.)

According to nutritionists, it's a combination of natural, complex carbohydrates such as fruits, brown rice, and whole-wheat breads, and proteins such as meats, eggs, fish, and dairy products, and fats that allows sugar to be slowly absorbed into the blood and a high-energy level to be maintained. When blood sugar stays high, the desperate craving for quick-sugar highs virtually disappears. This is why it's so important for dieters to abstain from sugar totally for a while, and eat satisfying, nutritious foods instead. Once you give up junk food, your sugar addiction will be no more, and if you do succumb every now and again, the junk will taste as false and empty—as well, junky

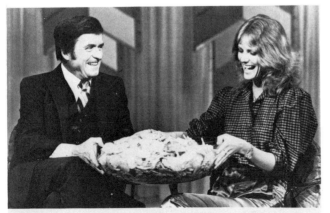

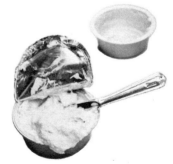

**PASS THE DIP**

When top model and television personality CHERYL TIEGS confides that she occasionally goes on a potato chip binge, MIKE DOUGLAS presents his cohost with a month's supply. CHERYL cohosts "THE MIKE DOUGLAS SHOW" on Friday, May 4 (Show # MD 0504/79) at _____ on channel _____.

—as it really is. When I was overweight I indulged in sweets constantly, but now I can confront an entire tray of French pastries and not even be tempted to touch one.

## THE BLOOD SUGAR EXPERIMENT

Let's try a simple experiment. The next time you feel starved at three in the afternoon, eat a candy bar. Note how rapidly you feel starved again. The following afternoon, eat a cup of unsweetened yogurt or drink a glass of skim milk. The sugar in milk—known as lactose—digests slowly, making you feel pleasantly full for a longer period of time, as you'll see for yourself.

Beware! Many breakfast cereals, packaged and canned goods, and even such unlikely foods as ketchup are loaded with sugar. A canned peach with a single tablespoon of syrup, for example, contains 3½ teaspoons of sugar. A bottle of Coca-Cola is one of the prime offenders in this department. Aside from minor things like making you tired, hungry, and fat, sugar can cause tooth decay, diabetes, hypoglycemia, and anxiety. Read the labels on the packages and cans and be on the lookout for the ones that contain sugar. Natural sugars such as honey and molasses are whole foods and therefore a little better for you than refined sugar is, but they, too, should be avoided.

## MIND OVER FODDER

As you know by now, no one understands better than I do how you lose all vestiges of self-control once that desire to eat overcomes you. You shake, sweat, feel "high." You don't stop to think about *why* you want to eat; you aren't thinking about your health or blood sugar; you're thinking only of how good that box of Mars bars or Mallomars is going to make you feel. Some food bingers inhale, gulp, and grab—they can't even wait till they get home to begin gorging themselves. Diet experts who advise you to "Grab a mate instead of a plate" aren't really allowing for the well-documented fact that the binger usually binges because he *has* no mate to grab (or the mate is ungrabbable).

Other bingers overeat out of habit; they fill the empty spaces in their day with the busy motion of lifting fork to mouth. I often overate because I was bored and had nothing much to think about. I thought about food, and thinking about food made me feel hungry, so I ate—and there we are.

Controlling and curing the binge syndrome isn't going to be easy. Don't underestimate the self-control you will need. It may help if you think of your over-eating as a *behavior* problem.

First, I recommend some soul-searching. When the desire to binge has you by the throat (the esophagus?), stop long enough to ask yourself, "Why am I about to eat ten gallons of maple walnut ice cream?" Think about the eating patterns of your childhood. Did your parents give you food as a reward, or when you felt cranky, sick, or sad? Did they used to punish you by sending you to bed without any dinner? Did they deny you dessert when you were "bad?" Most overeaters discover that food is associated for them with feelings of gratification or the lack of it. The main problem with using food to gratify yourself is that it doesn't do the job; you usually feel worse, not better, after con-suming all the goodies. And the pounds you gain are guaranteed to take the edge off any pleasure you might feel.

Try substituting other activities for overeating. Many people begin the chow-down the minute they get home from work. I automatically used to head straight for the fridge at 5:00 P.M. I discovered it helped to visit a friend on my way home, or to go shopping, or to attend an exercise class. If you binge mainly at a certain hour every day, plan a regular activity for that time slot. And *concentrate* on that activity, whether it's a course for credit or an escapist movie. If you're spending that time with friends, give all your attention to what they're saying. If food is offered, have only a glass of juice or a cup of tea. If you overeat because you feel lonely, volunteer some of your spare time at a worthwhile organization—hospital, orphanage, school.

There are now many clinics and diet clubs that deal professionally with the problem of overeating. Over-eaters Anonymous and the Weight Watchers' organi-zations have made dieting into a form of group therapy. They encourage their members to speak out about the feelings that led them to overeat, help them develop new habits and attitudes toward food, and provide all-important moral support. Chances are at least one of these organizations has a chapter in your area.

Don't forget that you are you and that the way you

choose to break your binging pattern must suit your personality. In an effort to stop stuffing themselves, some people have gone so far as to fantasize their favorite foods crawling with bugs, or to coat cakes with Tabasco sauce, or to get hypnotized. How you do it is up to you. The first step is to get yourself to do it!

## WILL AND WON'T POWER

Special menus, calorie counters, behavior modification plans, and soul-searching will be to no avail without the power to say a simple and emphatic "no" to food. When you're tempted to order a three-dip banana split, no advice, however well meant, will deter you; only the small, firm voice inside you can help. No one can give you that power to say no; you're going to have to find it for yourself and in yourself. You will probably say yes a good many times before you say no, but your desire to become thin, look good, and stay healthy and in control will doubtless win out in the end.

## C.T.'S MINUTE-TO-MINUTE GUIDE TO A SLIM FIGURE

I've listed some techniques that can be practiced all day long.

### The Morning Weigh-in

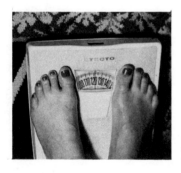

It takes the most courage to step on the dreaded scale the day after you've been particularly self-indulgent, because you may be able to fool yourself but the scale does not lie. As soon as you see that you've gained a pound, cut back on your food consumption. It's easier to get strict with yourself after you've gained a mere sixteen ounces than after you've gained ten pounds and your whole system is out of whack. I've become so aware of my body since I learned about good nutrition that I know when I've gained even before I set foot on the scale. That should be *your* goal, too. Meanwhile, weigh in every morning.

### Not Eating After Six

Whenever I feel that I'm gaining, that a pound or two may be gaining on *me*, I have an early supper and that's it, I don't let another morsel pass my lips after 6:00 P.M. This is a fail-proof way of removing extra pounds, because your body has time to burn up its daily calories before you go to sleep. And by not a morsel, I mean *nothing*. If you have plans to join friends for a late meal or if your husband is coming home late and expects dinner, have yours early and drink only a glass of wine at the table.

### Keeping a Food Diary

Write down the kind and amount of food you eat, the time of day you eat it, and how you feel. This diary will reveal your eating habits to you at the same time that it forces you to account for every bite you take. Most importantly, it will focus your mind on monitoring—and cutting down on—food consumption.

### Keeping It Up in Restaurants

Restaurants offer one tempting treat after another, serve large portions, lots of starches, divine desserts, and, in short, provide a matchless opportunity for you to relinquish—in one fell slurp—your slowly improving habits. Since, like most career women, I have to eat in restaurants fairly often, I've had to learn the art of restaurant resistance.

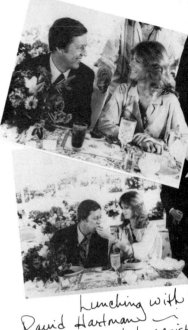

*Lunching with David Hartman— at first he tried to resist*

Sometimes I order a food I'm not particularly crazy about, like smoked salmon or antipasto, so I'm always sure to leave something on my plate. And even when I order my favorite foods, I try never to finish the portion the restaurant heaps onto the plate. If you feel guilty about leaving food on your plate, there is a delightfully unchic, very practical carrier known as the doggie bag. It's also a good idea to order a "healthy" food that you might never be inspired to prepare at home—something in the liver or kidney family, for instance, that's packed with vitamins. I always ask the waiter not to serve me potatoes, rolls, or creamed vegetables if they come with the meal. And if the entrée is served with lots of gravy or a rich sauce, I usually finesse that too. I sometimes order two appetizers and a soup instead of an entrée. I also make it a point to frequent Japanese, Chinese, and seafood restaurants that serve low-calorie fare, instead of Italian, French, and steakhouse restaurants. And when I order lunch from a coffee shop, I make my sandwich serve as instant diet fare by stripping off the top slice of bread—there's no need to eat a hamburger with both buns.

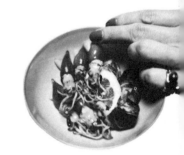

### Breakfast Binging

Though I am now just about indifferent to the sweets I craved when I was fat, I sometimes get that old urge for a piece of rich layer cake dripping with frosting. When this happens I try to hold off until breakfast, because if you have to eat something fattening, early morning is the best time to do it. You then have the whole day to burn off all the calories. Eating sweets after a big evening meal is the quickest way to pile on pounds. Cake for breakfast, needless to say, should be an infrequent indulgence for any diet-conscious woman. But then again, it's not every woman who can face a chocolate layer cake early in the morning.

### Beginning Your Diet with a Binge

Before you go on a serious diet, I recommend that you eat all the food you can manage for three solid days. The point is to overdo it, knowing that you will never overeat again. While you're stuffing yourself, take note of how your body is reacting, and form a cartoon mental picture of how all that junk that's now inside you is going to make you look. At the end of the three days, I guarantee that you will be looking forward to your diet.

### Substituting Quality for Quantity

In my diets at the end of this chapter, I recommend expensive delicacies such as smoked salmon, oysters, and exotic fruits. When you're eating less, you can afford high-quality foods. By cutting out ice cream, cake, soda, and lots of bread and meats, you save all around. If both you and your husband are overweight, buy small quantities of good cuts of filet mignon, instead of the large, cheaper cuts. And when you're lunching out, forget the Coca-Cola, french fries, and —ah!—cherry pie à la mode. Order a single dish such as lobster salad. The check will come to about the same.

### Visual Aides

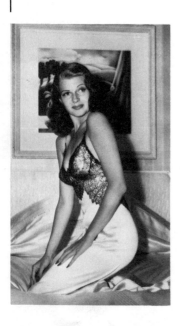

This is one of the oldest motivational tricks in the book—but a good one. The image of Rita Hayworth on the late show was the inspiration I once needed in order to begin a serious diet. I then went to the magazine stands and found examples of the best-maintained bodies. Overcoming embarrassment, and petty jealousy, I taped up these tear sheets all around my apartment. I was openly admitting to myself—and others—that there was a big discrepancy between me and the clippings I'd chosen to represent my far-off goal. Visual aides can also function as a weapon against temptation. Clip a picture of the figure you'd like to have and tack it up on the icebox door or on a full-length mirror. The mirror itself, of course, is by simple definition your most useful visual aide. Open your eyes and keep looking. Trying on a bikini in front of the mirror once a month is a good tell-me-no-lies way to check your progress.

### Packing a Snack

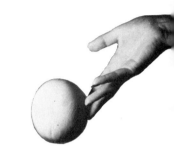

I feel hungry between meals or suffer gnawing hunger pangs whenever I have to miss or put off a meal. My blood sugar drops and I long for a good low-down calorie-loaded junk food orgy. I've learned to carry some low-calorie diversions in my tote bag, which someone, with good reason, once referred to as a snack pack. Oranges are the best—they give quick energy, taste great, and contain vitamins, too. If you pack a snack, make sure it's not some self-defeating and figure-defacing item like fudge brownies or chocolate-chip cookies.

### The Twenty-four-Hour Fast

When I need to drop a pound in a big hurry, I skip dinner, breakfast and lunch the next day, and eat a small dinner the following evening. This modified fast, believe it or not, is both safe and effective. Having skipped dinner, you wake up in the morning feeling light and energetic, and by lunchtime you're savoring the evening meal. This is one diet where you never feel "starved."

## MISTAKES PEOPLE MAKE

### Choosing the Wrong Diet

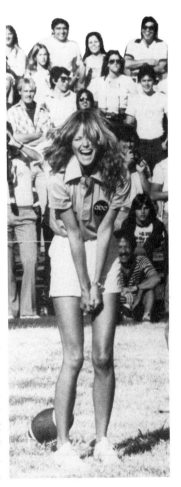

To maintain a slim figure you must develop sensible attitudes toward food and exercise. Many people recklessly embark on "miracle diets," featuring a small number of foods in odd, even bizarre, combinations, which supposedly help you burn off fat rapidly. A famous nutritionist, Carlton Fredericks, once quipped that the only thing miraculous about "miracle diets" is that people survive them. These diets are dangerous because the limited number of nutrients they provide eventually causes the body to take the nutrients it needs from its own cells. Beware of the following: the Atkins diet, which recommends high-calorie fats and no carbohydrates, is riskily high in cholesterol and

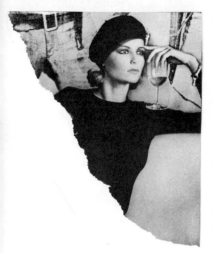

eliminates important nutrients; the Stillman diet, which has you eating an unlimited number of rich proteins and few carbohydrates and drinking eight glasses of water per day, may cause fatigue, nausea, and diarrhea; the macrobiotic diet, consisting mainly of brown rice, a few vegetables and fruits, and reduced fluids, when practiced in the extreme, may actually result in starvation; and the liquid protein diet, possibly the most dangerous of them all, is to be avoided at all costs without close medical supervision.

There are endless variations of these diets which I haven't mentioned. In general, the only really safe and effective way to diet is to eat both fewer calories and as many different foods as you can.

### Forgetting Liquids

Most of us on diets forget that liquids are food. Be sure to count the calories in liquids. A single Coca-Cola contains four or five teaspoons of solid sugar. Orange juice is good for quick energy and loaded with Vitamin C, but it's also loaded with calories. Alcohol, too, contains a great many calories. Next time you're at a party or your local bar, order a spritzer (half wine and half Perrier with a twist); it's refreshing and contains half the calories of one glass of wine. Or try two ounces of orange juice mixed with two ounces of mineral water for breakfast. If black coffee is too bitter for you, just add some skim milk. Quite aside from being bitter, it can make you jumpy and nervous—using up a lot of your energy at once, so I often substitute a cup of hot water with lemon juice, which, believe it or not, tastes pretty good. And instead of sweet colas, I usually ask for Perrier water with a slice of lime.

### Substituting Sweets

Diet soda is the mainstay of many dieters and I'm all for it. But "diet" sweets should be eaten sparingly if at all. On the whole they add up to more junk. When you're dieting, you should try and stay away from sweets of all kinds. Substitute fruit and low-calorie drinks for confections and soda.

### Gulping It Down

Diet experts believe almost to a man that if you eat your food too rapidly, your nervous system won't have time to warn you when you're full. Try to eat slowly. Lay down your fork between each bite, or chew longer, or take smaller bites. Don't read or watch TV while you eat or the amount you consume may get lost in the plot. *Concentrate* on what you're eating and on how good it tastes.

### Holding Back and Back and Back

There is a thin line between exercising the will power necessary to stay slim and totally depriving yourself of the foods you enjoy. If you never indulge yourself, life can seem rather grim. Once in a blue moon I treat myself to an enormous stack of pancakes complete with maple syrup, blueberries, bacon, sausages, and butter. Eating a small piece of cake once a week or so won't make you fat and may make you happy. When you're first dieting you should probably give up sweets altogether in order to kick the habit. And even after that, only occasional cravings should be indulged.

### Buying Foods You Shouldn't Even Be Thinking About

I refuse to have cakes, cookies, or even peanuts around the house. If you *really* want to avoid temptation, don't buy the stuff. Having to go all the way to the store to buy food that will only make you fat may make you think twice. Don't use children, husbands, or roommates as an excuse for stocking up; the things that pile the pounds on you and undermine your health do the same to them. And when you do buy a treat for your family or friends, buy enough for one time only.

## GET YOUR VITAMINS AND MINERALS THE NATURAL WAY

Vitamins stimulate cell growth and aid digestion and nerve function. They also help convert the food you eat into energy. Many people supplement their diets with vitamin and mineral pills in the belief that large random doses of supplements can preserve youth, cure all manner of ailments, and improve hair, skin, and nails. All well and good. But I make sure that the vitamins I take are prescribed by a nutritionist. Vitamin and mineral supplements should be approached with the greatest caution. A daily multi-vitamin pill is definitely a good idea, but no one should prescribe large amounts of vitamins or minerals for herself. Many nutritionists feel that not enough is known about the effect of large doses of vitamins on the human body; they cite that some vitamins in large

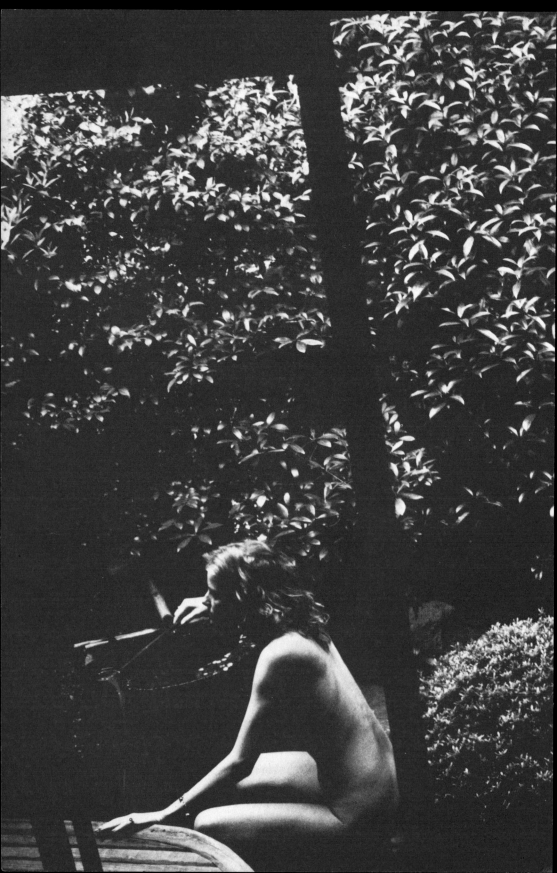

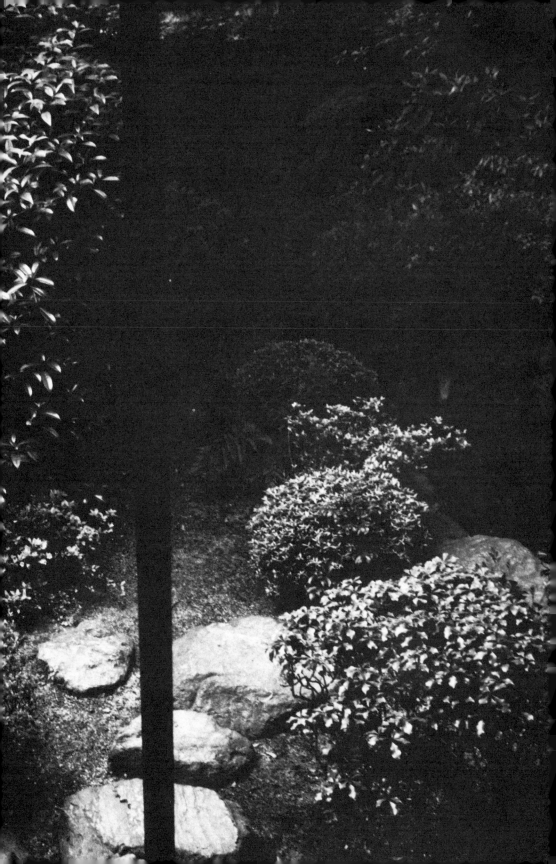

doses, such as Vitamins A and D, which are stored in the body, can be toxic. Overdoses of other vitamins can cause gastric disturbances, skin problems, and other damage. In most cases, as with Vitamin C, the body simply eliminates the excess vitamins—but why take a chance?

The best way to get vitamins and minerals is from natural foods. Some excellent sources, which can be taken as supplements, *are* foods and are easily absorbed by the body: brewer's yeast, wheat germ, kelp, raw bran. Here's a list of vitamins and some essential minerals, a description of how they affect your health and your appearance, and the names of some foods that contain them. Your best bet for good nutrition is to make sure that you regularly eat foods that have *all* these vitamins and minerals in them.

### Vitamin A

*What it does:* Improves vision; keeps skin smooth and hair and nails lustrous.

*Where to find it:* Green vegetables (spinach, broccoli, string beans); yellow vegetables (carrots, squash); apricots.

### Vitamin Bs

(There are many vitamins in the B family and few foods contain them all: $B_1$, $B_2$, $B_6$, $B_{12}$, biotin, choline, folic acid, inositol and PABA, and so on.)

*What they do:* Aid metabolism, growth, and the functions of internal organs, including the brain; reduce stress; help prevent excess oil in skin as well as skin discolorations.

*Where to find them:* Liver, brewer's yeast, bran, wheat germ, brown rice, bean curd, watercress, spinach, green leafy vegetables; eggs for Vitamin $B_{12}$.

### Vitamin C

*What it does:* Helps body resist infection; helps in preventing colds; improves teeth and gums; helps keep skin firm and elastic.

*Where to find it:* Citrus fruits, watercress, spinach, tomatoes, carrots.

### Vitamin D

*What it does:* Helps build bones and teeth.

*Where to find it:* Fish and enriched milk.

### Vitamin E

*What it does:* Improves skin; aids healing processes; and helps prevent blood clots.

*Where to find it:* Unrefined vegetable oils, liver, wheat germ, spinach, celery, watercress.

### MINERALS

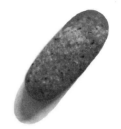

### Calcium

*What it does:* Helps build bones and teeth; aids blood clotting; reduces fatigue; fosters relaxation; helps prevent insomnia.

*Where to find it:* Milk (the richest source), watercress, spinach, carrots, salmon.

### Iodine

*What it does:* Regulates the functions of the thyroid gland, which regulates the functions of the entire body.

*Where to find it:* Shellfish, iodized salt, kelp, spinach, cranberries.

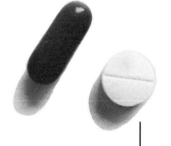

### Iron

*What it does:* Builds red blood corpuscles; carries oxygen to various parts of the body (women are often deficient in iron, and need to take a supplement, which works best when taken with Vitamin C).

*Where to find it:* Liver, eggs, whole grain breads or cereals, wheat germ, dried fruits, spinach, watercress.

### Magnesium

*What it does:* Synthesizes proteins in the body; protects nerves; prevents cramps.

*Where to find it:* Whole grains, spinach, green leafy vegetables.

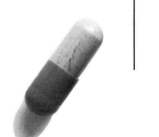

### Potassium

*What it does:* Gives muscles pliancy; aids nervous system, cell and tissue life.

*Where to find it:* Almost all fruits and vegetables; whole grains and nuts.

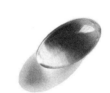

### Sodium (or salt)

*What it does:* Spurs digestive juices; helps eliminate carbon dioxide.

*Where to find it:* Spinach, watercress, whole grains,

seafood. (Too much salt can cause fluid retention, hypertension, and other problems. Try to lower your intake of table salt, and heighten the flavor of food with lemon juice and other condiments.)

Other minerals needed by the body are zinc, fluoride, copper, sulphur, and manganese, to name just a few.

You'll have noticed that I mentioned certain foods several times. Spinach and watercress contain virtually *all* the vitamins and minerals. Carrots, too, are rich in fiber and vitamins. Wheat germ, brewer's yeast, whole grains, and liver also double as nature's vitamin pills.

## C.T.'S TIME-SAVING, LIFE-SAVING, MONEY-SAVING DIET

I have never had any ambitions to be a gourmet. Nevertheless, food is very important to me. My career keeps me so busy I have no choice but to go for the most sensible foods, which also happen to be the most nourishing and the easiest to prepare.

The recipes that follow require minimal time in the kitchen. Even the big bow-wow gourmet cooks I know don't want to do it every day of the week.

The foods I've chosen will keep you supplied with all the nutrients you need for health and vitality and at the same time amount to a good basic diet. If you eat a Cheryl Tiegs breakfast, lunch, and dinner (as yet served in no restaurants I've heard of), you will be consuming only 1200 calories a day or thereabouts. If you want to take in fewer calories, just cut down on the margarine, butter, or oils, but never eliminate all the fats in your diet—they nourish the skin and hair with necessary oils and help burn up those calories.

I provide a *selection* of breakfasts, lunches, and dinners, instead of the rigid Monday-through-Sunday calendar of meals. That way you can decide what you want to eat and when. My menus are only suggestions; your eating habits should reflect *your* personality as mine do mine. Maybe that's why these meal suggestions feature some foods and combinations of foods that the regular diets don't include.

## BREAKFAST

Nutritional studies have shown that people who eat a high-protein breakfast, in combination with some carbohydrates and fat, work with greater efficiency and feel better throughout the day; their blood sugar level stays high. I wouldn't dream of skipping breakfast.

### C.T.'s Favorite

4 oz. unsweetened orange juice (for quick energy) = 55 calories
1 bran muffin (provides a solid carbohydrate for long-lasting energy and fiber) = 106 calories
1 teaspoon margarine (select a margarine made from pure vegetable oil) = 34 calories
1 cup plain yogurt (provides protein, calcium, and bacterial organisms to aid digestion) = 150 calories
1 cup hot water spiked with lemon juice

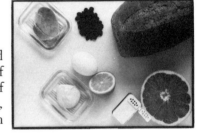

Total calories = 345

### C.T.'s Mock Eggs Benedict
(A Slimming Version of the Calorific Treat)

½ grapefruit sprinkled with cinnamon = 50 calories
Tea or coffee
Mock Eggs Benedict = 310 calories
    To make C.T.'s M.E.B., top a piece of thin-sliced whole wheat or pumpernickel toast with 1 ounce of boiled ham. Poach or boil an egg and place on top of ham. Top with 1 tablespoon lemon mayonnaise, which you make by beating 2 tablespoons of lemon juice into ¼ cup mayonnaise.

Total calories = 360

### C.T.'s Quick Blender Milkshake

My favorite way to quickly fill up on high-quality calories.
1 cup skim milk = 90 calories
1 banana (bananas are particularly rich in potassium) = 100 calories
½ cup orange juice = 55 calories
1 egg = 75 calories
1 teaspoon honey (optional) = 20 calories
    Put above ingredients into blender jar and blend till smooth. For fewer calories, you can add just a bit of banana or dispense with it altogether. You can also substitute a vegetable-based protein powder for the egg. You can even drink this breakfast as you're running out the door.

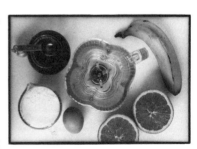

Total calories = 340

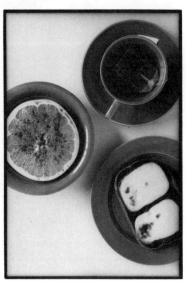

### C.T.'s "G.M.A." G.C. (or "Good Morning America" Grilled Cheese)

Most people think of a grilled cheese as luncheon fare, but it also makes a quick and nutritious breakfast. For the morning, I prefer one of the lighter cheeses such as mozzarella.

*½ grapefruit sprinkled with cinnamon and broiled = 50 calories*

*1 piece thin-sliced rye or whole wheat bread = 55 calories*

*2 oz. skim milk mozzarella cheese (¼ of an 8 oz. package) = 160 calories*

*½ teaspoon margarine = 17 calories*

Spread the bread with margarine, top with mozzarella, and broil until the cheese is melted and browned. Broil grapefruit at the same time.

*Total calories = 282*

### C.T.'s Oriental Pudding

Dieters often crave a sweet in the morning but doughnuts and Danishes are taboo, because they provide only useless calories. I've discovered that a bland-tasting Oriental food called tofu, or bean curd, which has few calories and is loaded with protein and the B vitamins, can be transformed into an energizing sweet, with the help of a little honey and flavoring. This breakfast has to be made the night before.

*1 block tofu (widely available in health-food or Oriental specialty stores) 120 grams of tofu or about 4 ounces = 86 calories*

*1 tablespoon honey (add an extra tablespoon if you're not dieting) = 60 calories*

*¼ cup skim milk = 22 calories*

Simmer bean curd in a pan of water for five minutes. Put bean curd, honey, and milk in a blender jar and add vanilla or almond flavoring to taste. Blend till smooth. Pour in a small bowl and sprinkle with cinnamon. Chill. This breakfast sweet is guaranteed to keep you satisfied till lunch.

*Total calories = 168*

### C.T.'s Quick Grab

You may be in too much of a rush to even think of breakfast and make the mistake of settling for a calorific treat from the coffee wagon. But there are nourishing breakfasts you can literally grab on your way out the door that will provide you with far more energy—and fewer calories. Let's grab:

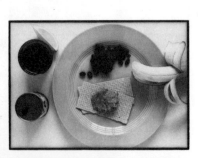

1. A *banana (filling, nutritious, and sweet) = 100 calories*
2. *Two slices of any whole-grain flatbread = approximately 50 calories, depending on brand. If you have time, divide 1 tablespoon peanut butter (rich in protein but very fattening) between them = 100 calories*
3. *A handful of raisins (lots of iron) = 112 calories*
4. *Eight ounces tomato juice = 50 calories, or 6 ounces orange juice = 75 calories; with two heaping tablespoons brewer's yeast mixed in = 60 calories. This is one of the most nutritious breakfasts grabbable. Yeast is one of our best natural sources of protein and the B vitamins. Warning: Many people are put off by the taste, so try different brands (available in health food stores) till you find one you like.*

## LUNCH

### C.T.'s Scandinavian Smorgasbord

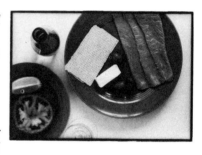

*2 ounces Nova Scotia smoked salmon (expensive and delicious) = 200 calories*
*1 ounce Neufchâtel cheese (less caloric than cream cheese) = 100 calories*
*2 slices Swedish flatbread = 50 calories*
*1 raw tomato = 25 calories*
*3 olives = 25 calories*
*1 glass of mineral water with 1 slice of lime and/or herbal tea sweetened with cinnamon and orange peel*

*Total calories = 400*

### C.T.'s Bunless Burger

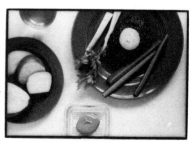

The all-American hamburger is fattening to begin with, and when you stuff it between two buns or slices of bread it becomes a big problem. The hamburger is just about everybody's favorite, however, and it's so quick and easy to prepare. I suggest treating it as if it were a mini-steak. Grill a 4-ounce hamburger made of ground round and add ½ teaspoon of a good-quality mustard, a thin strip of Roquefort cheese, and 1 teaspoon chutney for zest. You can also mix chopped onions and parsley into the meat before grilling it.
*1 bunless burger = 195 calories*
*Tomato, celery, and pepper sticks = 50 calories*
*Unsweetened beverage*
*1 apple, peach, pear, or nectarine = 100 calories*

*Total calories = 345*

### C.T.'s Vitamin Pill

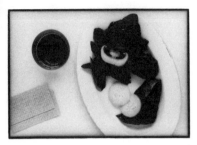

This contains so many vitamins and minerals it amounts to a substitute for a multi-vitamin pill. It's a good lunch to eat before going on that twenty-four-hour fast I suggested. And if you hate liver, no problem—simply substitute a glass of brewer's yeast and tomato juice.

*1 cup spinach salad (fresh raw spinach, carefully washed) = 50 calories*
*1 tablespoon oil and vinegar dressing with ½ teaspoon mustard = 120 calories*
*2 slices Swedish flatbread = 50 calories*
*2 ounces sautéed calf's liver = 118 calories*
*Herbal tea*

*Total calories = 338*

Note: If you want only salad for lunch, increase the amount of spinach and dressing, add a chopped hard-boiled egg, raw mushrooms, and a slice of bacon, and Violà!

### C.T.'s No-Mayo Fish Salad

There's no rule that says fattening mayonnaise has to be a feature of a fish salad. Substitute yogurt and flavor the salad with chopped scallions or chives, fresh dill or parsley, chopped olives and celery and lemon juice. Come on, use your imagination!

*1 cup water-packed crab, tuna, or lobster salad made with yogurt = approximately 130 calories*
*Cucumber salad (sliced cucumber with 1 tablespoon dressing) = 140 calories*
*Unsweetened beverage*

*Total calories = 270*

### "I Hate Cottage Cheese"

I've always associated bland cottage cheese with a deprivation diet. Instead, I use the Italian cheese ricotta, which looks a little like cottage cheese but has a richer texture and tastes delicious. Ricotta is higher in calories, so you'll just have to eat less. If you are seriously dieting and feel duty-bound to spring for cottage cheese in a restaurant, sprinkle it with chives and fresh ground pepper to make it a bit more exciting.

*½ cup skim-milk ricotta = 125 calories*
*2 slices Swedish flatbread = 50 calories*
*6 olives = 50 calories*
*1 slice cantaloupe or honeydew melon = 30 calories per quarter-slice melon*
*Italian espresso, or tea*

*Total calories = 255*

## C.T.'s Instant Satisfaction

My favorite lunch is the one I find waiting for me in the refrigerator already prepared. Among other things, it saves me the expense and temptation of eating in a restaurant. How about:

*2 ounces cheese (Mysöst, Edam, or mozzarella, which are lower in calories than the heavier, oily cheeses such as Cheddar and Brie); or 2 small slices cold turkey, chicken, or roast beef; or 2 hard-boiled eggs = approximately 200 calories*
*Celery, carrot, pepper, or cucumber sticks = 50 calories*
*1 whole tomato = 25 calories*
*1 small can tomato or vegetable juice = 50 calories*
*2 slices flatbread = 50 calories*
*A piece of fruit = 100 calories*

*Total Calories = 475*

## DINNER

Who doesn't enjoy relaxing over a home-cooked meal in the evening? Dinner is the most important meal of the day for me, and I like to make it a festive occasion, with good, simple-to-prepare dishes and candlelight. Because I feel wine adds a great deal, I've included it —calories or no calories—in almost all my dinner menus.

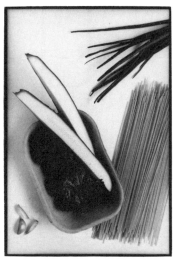

### Spaghetti Diet-Style

Pasta is not a total write-off for dieters, because small amounts are low in calories.
*1 cup tender spaghetti = 155 calories*
*¼ cup each broccoli and zucchini = 25 calories*
*2 tablespoons olive oil = 250 calories*
*Chopped garlic and scallions*
   Sauté garlic and scallions in oil, then add broccoli and zucchini. Cook only a couple of minutes; the vegetables should be crisp. Spoon over the cooked spaghetti.
*1 glass white wine = 70 calories*
*½ cup raspberries or blueberries topped with 1 tablespoon yogurt = 60 calories*

*Total calories = 560*

### Baked Fish

*1 average serving baked fish = approximately 250 calories depending on type of fish and size of portion*
   Buy a whole fish such as trout, bluefish, or flounder, or use a fillet of sole. Melt 1 teaspoon butter in ¼ cup dry vermouth and pour over raw fish. Sprinkle with

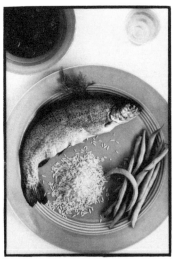

dill. Bake in 400° oven till fish is tender and white when pierced with a fork (approximately fifteen minutes). Baste once or twice while cooking. Serve with one slice of lemon.

*1 cup steamed string beans mixed with ¼ cup mushrooms sautéed in 1 teaspoon margarine = 75 calories*
*½ cup brown rice = 50 calories*
*1 glass white wine = 70 calories*
*½ cup fruit compote flavored with 1 teaspoon sherry = 65 calories*

*Total calories = 510*

### Easy-Does-It Vegetarian

This is my adaptation of a lunch served at the "21" Club in New York.
*1 cup fresh mushrooms = 15 calories*
*1 cup spinach = 20 calories*
*1 cup chopped broccoli = 45 calories*
*1 cup bean sprouts, optional = 25 calories*
*1 chopped scallion*
*1 tablespoon peanut or sesame oil = 100 calories*
  Heat oil in skillet or Chinese wok. Sauté scallions. Add broccoli, bean sprouts, mushrooms, and spinach, and stir fry for several minutes till tender. You can also steam the vegetables.
*Top with a poached egg = 75 calories*
*Serve with ½ cup brown rice = 50 calories*
*½ small papaya = 40 calories*
*Tea*

*Total calories = 370*

### Chicken Little

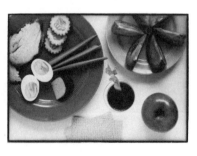

Chicken is very nutritious, lean, and easily digested. It's also rich in calcium, phosphorus and iron. My favorite part of the chicken, if you really want to know, is the skin, but if you're dieting, definitely forget about that part. Chicken goes well with so many seasonings and flavors. Try basting it with lemon juice and powdered ginger or soy sauce, or sprinkling it with tarragon before broiling.

*4 ounces cranberry juice (good for your kidneys) = 75 calories*
*½ small boned chicken or Cornish game hen, which is tenderer and more elegant (3½ ounces of chicken meat contain 171 calories)*
*Endive, watercress, and sliced water chestnut salad with 1 tablespoon oil and vinegar dressing = 160 calories*

1 small baked squash (any variety) with ½ teaspoon
   butter = 100 calories
Tea

Total calories = approx. 506

### Salad à la C.T.

I truly love preparing a giant salad, which brings out
whatever dormant and long-buried "gourmet instincts" I may have. Served with flatbread or bread-
sticks, the following salad makes a very nice light
dinner. You can use any or all of the ingredients I've
listed below, or improvise as you go along—you can
put almost anything in a salad (apart from endangered
species!) and it'll still taste good.

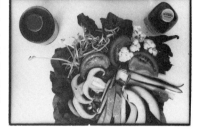

1 cup arugula or spinach leaves
1 cup Boston lettuce
Bean sprouts
Thin strips of boiled ham or turkey
Radishes
Tomato
Pepper
Avocado
Thin slices of cucumber or raw zucchini
Sliced raw mushrooms
Raw cauliflower buds
¼ cup sunflower seeds
2 tablespoons dressing of your choice (if you make a
   large salad for several people, serve dressing in a
   gravy boat so dieters can measure their portion with
   a tablespoon)

Food is primarily life-sustaining but we do *not* live
by sustenance alone, and food can even be as much a
form of therapy as therapy itself. The ritual places for
eating range from our own homes to the drive-in and
diner, to the restaurant glistening with the apparatus
of French cuisine, to the little bistro for the couple
just out of college and not yet expense-accounted for,
to the high-powered, business-oriented, status-based
lunch club. But whatever the ambience, whatever the
cost, one's devotion to one's own mouth and stomach
is finally relentless.

Since food plays such an important role in our sense
of well-being and warm connection to the world, we
must try to take advantage of the three opportunities
a day we have for food therapy.

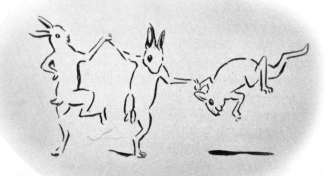

# 4

# Push Pull, Push Pull: The High Road to Muscle Tone

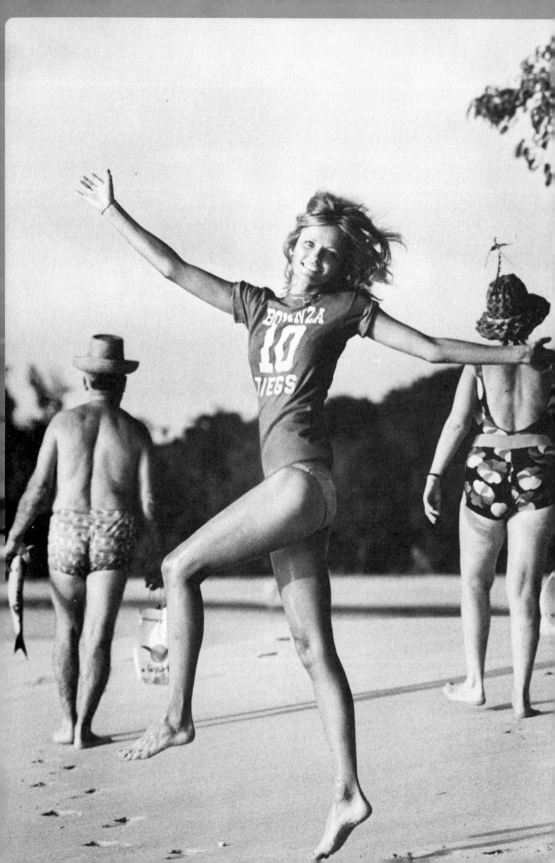

*A* good body has to be a whole lot more than just thin. (A thin body can be formless, slack, and even flabby.) The arms and legs should be muscular, the abdomen flat and firm, the back strong and well-toned: the good body should look like it can't wait to get moving at a good trot, can't wait to run, jump, and bend. A lithe figure makes a terrific impression: the person who possesses it is someone who is obviously on the side of life, someone who has learned how to live the healthy, active way. I say "learned" because it's no trick, and it's not luck.

Few women are born with perfectly proportioned bodies, but every woman, even the roundest of the round, can achieve the best version of the figure she has—by exercising. Being a great big beefy glob is the same as being a parasite; deep down, you have the distinct feeling—and if you don't, there's probably a small, nagging voice that tells you you should—that you're adding nothing to the world but your own weight. And every day, the idea of getting out of yourself becomes harder and harder to contemplate. But take heart: you don't have to be stuck with this indulgent self. You have only one life to live—and none of us gets out of it alive, right?—so you might as well go all the way with it, get the most you can out of it, lift your sights a little higher. All you have to do is make an effort, and if you aren't a natural athlete, what you can do is exercise. Oh I know, everybody has some brisk excuse or other for *not* exercising. It's so easy to wallow around—and just roll down jelly-roll lane—but it's such a waste of precious time.

Exercise alone will not make you fit any more than dieting by itself will make you shapely. So take a good deep breath and decide to do both!

If you're the right weight for your body frame, and still notice sags, bulges, and other gloomy annexes on your silhouette, then your body is clearly famished for exercise.

If you'll get into a bathing suit and be seated, Dr. Tiegs will be with you in a few minutes. Now: with your bathing suit on, stand in front of a full-length mirror. Take a good look at the whole of you. Odds are you are not faultlessly shaped and that your vanity has just been stung, if not demolished. Console your-

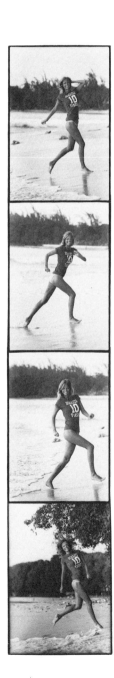

self with the thought that none of us looks like her dream picture of herself. And now I'm going to pester you with some questions. Answer them truthfully—if you don't, it's like lying to your shrink, you'll wind up cheating only yourself.

■ *Do your arms have enough muscles in them to form curves? Raise one arm to shoulder height: is there flab on the underside of the upper arm?*

■ *Stretch your leg out in front of you and lift it about a foot off the ground. Now feel the muscles in your upper thighs with your fingers. Or are they non-existent?*

■ *Turn your profile to the mirror. Stand up straight. Now look at your lower abdomen. Does your stomach feel mooshy instead of firm when you press it with your fingers?*

■ *Look closely at your shoulders. Is one of them hunched up, slouched over, or what?*

■ *Stretch up toward the ceiling with your hands. Then, with your knees perfectly straight and your feet a few inches apart, bend down and try to touch your toes. You can't?*

■ *Do you have those glumps of fat jocularly referred to as "riding breeches" on the outside of your thighs even though your weight is close to what it should be? Do you also sport the curdled flesh they call "cellulite?"*

■ *Are your hands and feet usually cold?*

■ *When you run up a flight of stairs, are you breathless?*

■ *Do you often feel "run down," even after a good night's sleep?*

You've just died a little, because you probably had to answer "yes" to most of these questions. I once had to.

And now back to what you have just seen for yourself in that full-length mirror.

A raised shoulder is often a sign of tension reflected in the alignment of your body. Weak muscles tense up easily, as do any muscles we hold in a distorted position for any length of time. And if we spend many hours at a desk or bent over a typewriter, the area around the shoulders and neck is almost certain to be tense and unaligned. Other obvious signs of body tension are tight, compressed lips and squinty eyes. Exercise creates flexibility in the muscles and joints; and the harder we work at it, the more effectively it relaxes us.

Women tend to pile up fat in the tissue of their buttocks, thighs, and arms. If your weight is near normal and still you are saddled with "riding breeches," your body is probably high in fat. "Cellulite" is the fancy term for fat deposits on those parts of your body that get little circulation—like buttocks and thighs, not to name names. We sit on "cellulite," and it bubbles under the pressure—not audibly but visibly, becoming in time dimpled and rough. Luckily, cellulite responds to the increased circulation that is one of the by-products of exercise.

If your hands and feet feel chilly in reasonably warm weather and icy when it's merely cold out, you are probably not receiving a strong enough flow of blood from your circulatory system. Exercise steps up the circulation, sends a warm greeting to hands and feet. After I've done my calisthenics, I can feel my fingers tingling, and it's an honest-to-God *alive* sensation, a reward for all my exertions.

If you do eat properly and you do get enough rest and you still feel fatigued, not even capable of true relaxation, then you are probably not aware of:

## WHAT EXERCISE CAN DO FOR YOU

### Improve the Function of Your Cardiovascular System

When you exercise vigorously, you are forcing your heart to work harder, beat faster. The heart is a muscle like any other, and the well-exercised heart can all the more easily cope with unusual exertions, such as shoveling snow after a storm. It pumps more blood—more quickly—through your veins, blood vessels, and arteries, thus toning and burnishing your whole system. In the process, all your internal organs receive a greater supply of nourishing plasma and oxygen at the same time that they are purged of impurities such as carbon dioxide. Before you know it, you're feeling less languid. The color and texture of your skin improve with exercise; blemishes fade out, fade away. Do you know when I look my best? After I've run around a tennis court for about an hour! To me, the natural glow that I feel at that time is more satisfying than any blusher or rouge could ever be. Running, sweating, and working off excess water, I feel as if I'm in ardent pursuit of whoever I have it in me to become.

## Improve Your Posture, Balance, and Coordination

Exercise strengthens and stretches the muscles in your back, shoulders, neck, and abdomen. The result is you hold your head higher, your spine straighter; your stomach is flatter, and your shoulders, for once, are sitting back and down. And if that isn't incentive enough, have you ever thought how standing up straight is the best way to reveal the lines of a beautiful outfit? And have you ever considered how—just maybe—slumping around with your feet splayed out is not the very best way to "win friends and influence people?"

Sports, modern dance, and ballet will put you on the road to balance and coordination, a road that from now on you will travel without bulging bags. People who do regular exercise move with more self-assurance and elegance; they have greater linear expression and more grace—because they understand their bodies, and they understand the space *around* their bodies. And moving with confidence is the first step to moving sensually, which as we all know works better than any dress or perfume yet invented.

## Increase Your Flexibility

A well-toned, flexible body is far less susceptible to accidents. Exercise points up the areas of your body that are stiff and weak. Once when I was doing deep knee bends in an exercise class, I experienced quite a shock: my ankles were about ready to give out—in any case, they gave out a warning crackle from deep within my ankle crust. If I hadn't done that exercise, I would never have thought about my ankles—I mean, why would anyone ever think about their ankles?—until I sprained one! So stand warned: weak, inflexible joints are easy to twist, even easier to break.

If your body is fit and nimble, you can perform physical tasks you might have assumed were way beyond your power of endurance. Last year, when ABC-TV sent me to Africa to host a special on Kenya,

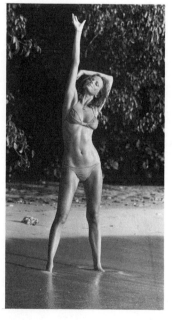

"Chin up, feet on the ground, keep reaching for the stars."

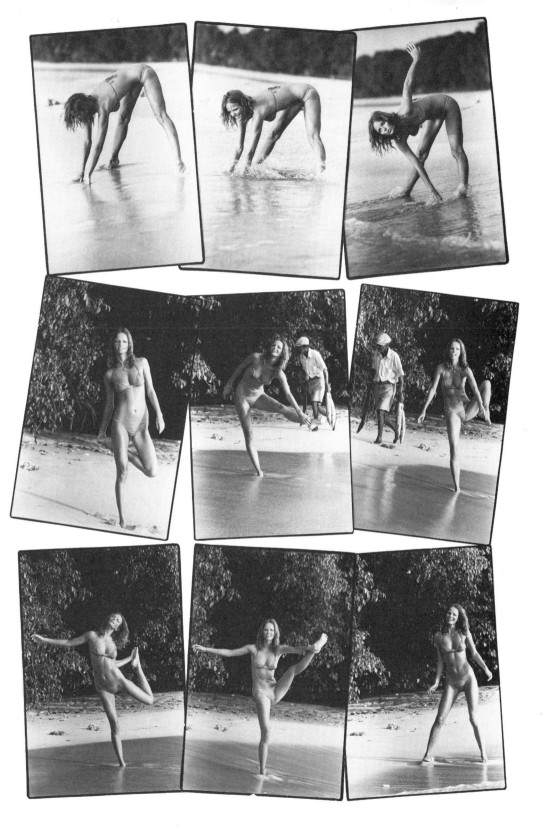

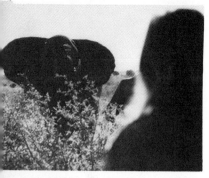

I suddenly found myself on the verge of being overtaken by a demonstrating, rampaging elephant herd (that's twenty thousand pounds I'm talking about!) in the volcanic lava fields of Tsavo National Park. I hesitate to think what might have happened to the special (and, parenthetically, to *me*) if I hadn't been in good enough shape to run for my life. As they say in Nairobi, *Shauri ya naungu*.

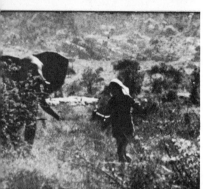

### Increase Your Mental Energy

When I'm in New York working under terrific pressure and not getting my usual exercise fix, I get much more irritable than I do in open-aired, even-tempered California. Fatigue, we now know, is more often the result of tension and pressure than of any job itself. The great upheavals take place inside us almost before we know it, and anxiety settles in our muscles as well as our minds. But one swift game of tennis or steamy session of calisthenics and you can feel as refreshed as if you'd just had eight hours of riftless sleep. And by the way, while exercise is supplying you with greater energy reserves and thus helping you stay more alert, it's also helping you sleep better. Few people who do regular exercise are insomniacs, since exercise dissipates the tension that during the day makes you feel part of the Living Dead—dull and dull-at-heart—and that during the night keeps you tossing, turning, and roving.

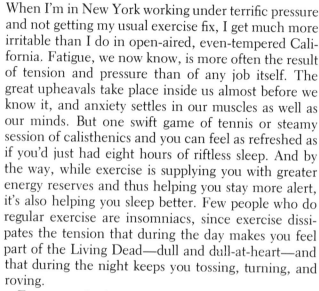

Everyone who has ever exercised systematically can vouch for the fact that a good run, swim, or game of squash is just about the best antidote for feeling "down." Exercise provides a release for pent-up feelings of depression, restlessness, and boredom. You get that ebullient feeling that, no matter what else, you have a strong, healthy body under your control.

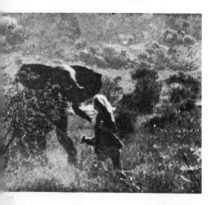

### Stifle and Depress an Enlarged Appetite

All the experts agree that nutrition and exercise go hand-in-hand: when you exercise, your body uses nutrients to create muscle cells. Studies have shown that truly vigorous exercise keeps the appetite at bay, especially in chronic overeaters. If you're someone who eats out of boredom or restlessness, why not substitute a little exercise at the times when you are tempted to raid the fridge.

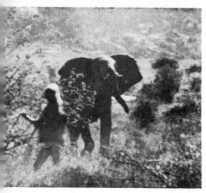

# FINDING THE RIGHT EXERCISE

To get all you can out of working out, you will very likely have to take up more than one kind of exercise. If you want to improve the functioning of heart, lungs, and circulatory system, then do an "aerobic" exercise —an activity that makes your heart beat faster and your lungs work harder, such as running, jumping rope, swimming, or playing a hard game of tennis, handball, or squash. While you do any one of these exercises your body will be consuming more oxygen, your blood pressure may well be reduced, and certainly your overall endurance will increase.

Aerobic exercise, however, is not enough to tone and strengthen all the muscles in your body. Any woman who wants a flat stomach and willowy waist will have to practice calisthenic exercises as well— spot-toning exercises, gymnastics, yoga. This stretch-tone-and-relax kind of exercise trims and shapes the parts of your body that aerobic exercise doesn't get to. (The body is a riddle—a very stylish one, to be sure— and riddles take solving.) Jogging, for example, shapes your thighs and calves, but does very little for your arms. The most complete-unto-itself aerobic exercise is swimming; it gives your chest, back, and legs a fine workout. Calisthenics relax your body and make it more flexible. In fact, if you're out of shape, you should limber up with a calisthenic exercise *before* attempting a vigorous sport; otherwise, you're just courting strains and sprains.

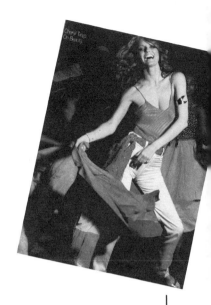

Let's say you've never exercised regularly in your life. Then your first job will be to choose an exercise you can stay with and even get to enjoy. This is a lot harder than it sounds, since if you're out of shape, almost any exercise is going to feel like some exotic torture and—at least at first—look like a bad dumb-show. As soon as you come up against all those un-fledged, unflexed muscles, each one of which is crying out to you, "Enough already!", you're going to want to abandon whatever exercise you've chosen. But stick with it. I believe in giving anything—from sitting down on up—a serious try.

Which isn't to say that I haven't pulled the plug on various activities I've taken up. I went through a jump-ing-rope-in-hotel-rooms phase while I was "on the road." I've jogged down more city streets than I can count in more cities than I can name. I've run in place like a little hamster, done sit-ups *beyond* number *before*

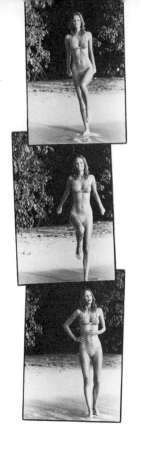

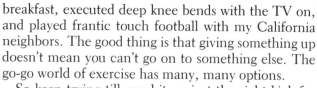

breakfast, executed deep knee bends with the TV on, and played frantic touch football with my California neighbors. The good thing is that giving something up doesn't mean you can't go on to something else. The go-go world of exercise has many, many options.

So keep trying till you hit on just the right kick for you. Waterskiing is exhilarating and phenomenal exercise—you get to cover a lot of ground (well, not ground exactly), see all the sights, splash all your friends, take a few death-defying chances, and benefit from an intense workout at one and the same time. But my heart belongs to tennis. To me there's nothing more delicious than slipping into a T-shirt and a pair of shorts (as opposed to stuffing myself into ski equipment or scuba gear) and getting a chance to utilize my competitive drive and sense of strategy.

Whatever exercise you wind up choosing, just remember that you have to practice it regularly and that it's not a bad idea if you learn to enjoy it. I've put together this list of pros and cons for the most popular types of exercise.

### Jogging

*What it can do for you:* Improve your cardiovascular system and your overall endurance; shape your legs; firm and raise your buttocks. No special equipment needed. A good calorie burner (ten to thirteen calories per minute!).

*What it can do to you:* Jogging can cause muscle strains, pulls, tendinitis, shin splints and other athletic injuries. If you're over thirty-five or generally out of shape, take it real slow at first. After about twelve minutes, alternate jogging with brisk walking. Jog on grass or dirt, preferably on a low-pollution day, and keep those hands and shoulders relaxed.

### Swimming

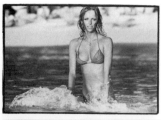

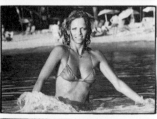

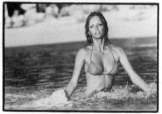

*What it can do for you:* Improve your cardiovascular system; exercise every major muscle group in your body, including your back and abdominal muscles; burn off calories at a particularly high rate, especially if the swimming is strenuous (thirty yards or more a minute). Places no stress on any one part of the body. Produces that heady combination of relaxation and invigoration. Particularly beneficial to the elderly and out of shape. But don't just swim, take your swimming seriously, swim energetically, keeping those arms and legs moving. Flutter kick with your legs straight but relaxed—the kicking motion originating from the hip, not the knee. So good-bye, torpor!

*What it can do to you:* Swimming in a chlorinated pool may irritate sinuses and dehydrate skin or dry hair, so make sure that afterwards you shower with soap and rinse all the pool water out of your hair. And, by the way, don't go and drown.

### Bicycling

*What it can do for you:* Strengthen your cardiovascular system; firm up your calf, thigh and back muscles. Cycle fast and maintain speed to get the best results; cycling on hilly terrain is ideal.

*What it can do to you:* Create tension in your neck and shoulders; put extra stress on your knee, hip, and ankle joints. But this is no time to be fastidious. As Tallulah Bankhead used to say, "Press on!"

### Jumping Rope

*What it can do for you:* Same benefits as jogging. A big plus is that you can jump rope indoors in a small area. Begin by jumping fifty times, alternating your feet as if you were running. Gradually work your way up to five hundred skips (at which time you'll explode in an asthmatic puff of dust). You'll need a seven-to-ten-foot cord, a good pair of sneakers, and a good sense of the absurd.

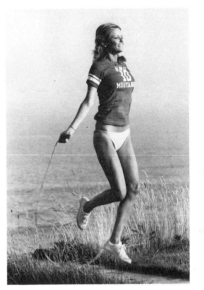

### Squash and Racquetball

*What they can do for you:* Utilize the main muscle group in your body; condition your cardiovascular system (though not quite as much as jogging and swimming can). Competitive sports benefit you the most, because all negative emotions get released in the course of the short, rippling life of the game.

### Skiing

*What it can do for you:* Improve your cardiovascular system (cross-country skiing—not downhill skiing, unless you do it for a long time); burn a fantastic fifteen to seventeen calories per minute.

*What it can do to you:* Kill you—the end of the day when the light fades and your furious energy uncoils is the time to be extra careful: that's when most accidents happen.

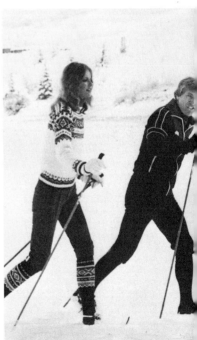

*with Bob "Beats" Beatt*

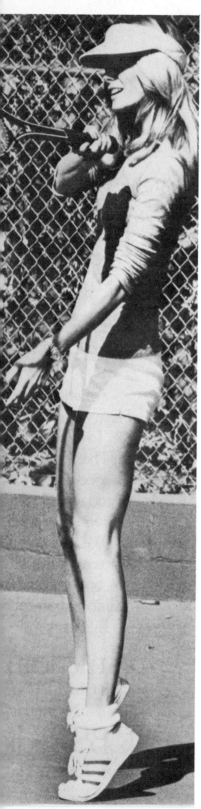

### Tennis Anyone?

*What it can do for you:* Strengthen your legs and your cardiovascular system (in a fast match you do about six miles' worth of running); provide an outlet for aggressive emotions; improve your coordination, balance, and overall endurance; uncramp your style.

### Calisthenics

*What they can do for you:* Help flexibility and muscle tone; "burn" fat in those out-of-the-way areas of your body; condition you for demanding aerobic activities and sports. For the best results, don't do calisthenics in fragments, and do them regularly.

### Yoga

*What it can do for you:* Make stiff, out-of-shape bodies flexible by stretching and relaxing your muscles; give you a sense of peace, of calm emotion; improve the function of your internal organs. Should be learned under proper supervision for maximum benefit and minimum strain.

*What it cannot do for you:* Condition your cardiovascular system.

### WHEN? HOW OFTEN? HOW MUCH?

Once is not enough! To see and feel any real results, you should exercise three or four times a week. And don't wait more than thirty-six hours between sessions, or your muscles will contract again and you'll forfeit some of the progress you've made. Do you really want to flatten your stomach and slim down your thighs? Then you've just got to spot exercise these treacherous areas as often as once a day.

Here I am preaching about the benefits of exercise (don't get me wrong, I truly believe in them and live by them), but I often wake up in the morning with a million ready-made reasons why I shouldn't have to move, let alone do calisthenics. I humor myself with, "I was up so late last night," or "I've been working so hard lately I really *deserve* an extra hour in bed," and of course there's always Scarlet O'Hara's inexpungible line about "tomorrow." In that smoked-brown-glassy-gloomy state between sleeping and waking, exercise looms up as an abnormal practice, a downright unnatural act. I've discovered that a few bleary-eyed sit-ups or push-ups while I'm still exquisitely under the covers are enough to get me tumbling out of bed in a rush of ease. If that isn't achieving a kind of oneness with yourself, I'd like to know what is.

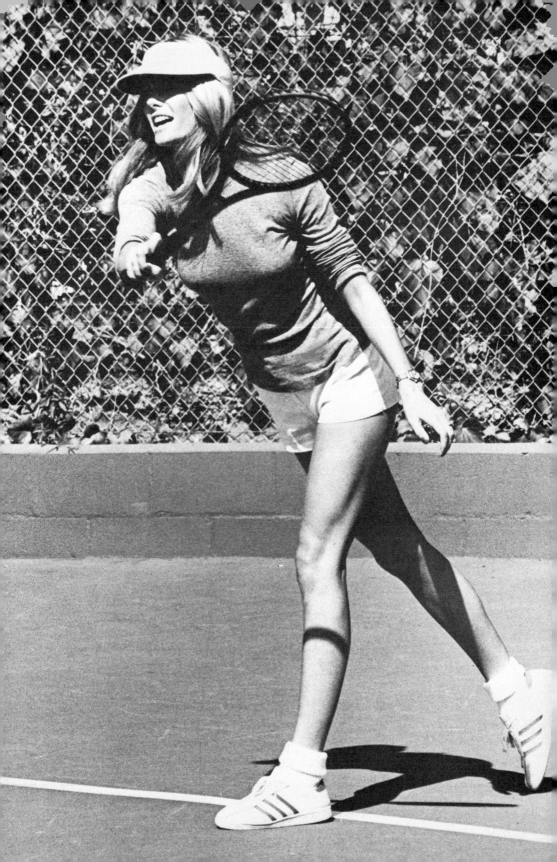

# HOW TO ENJOY THE TREADMILL

The main thing is to think of whatever exercise you've chosen to practice in bright, spangled terms. Exercise should be a challenging part of your day, not just a time-consuming medicine to keep your body from disintegrating before your very eyes. Here are some suggestions for making exercise more fun.

### Wear a Beautiful Exercise Outfit

Leotards and tights are now available in shimmery, synthetic fabrics (Lycra and nylon) and cheerful colors. I have a drawerful, and just looking at them inspires me. Jogging suits also come in a variety of attractive fabrics and designs, and even jogging shoes are now full of life. Dressing as if there were a real pleasure in store for you when you exercise will boost your morale. There's a lot to be said for pleasant associations.

### Call for Madder Music

When you're doing calisthenics or yoga, jumping rope, or just jogging in place, it's usually a good idea to play some Baroque Fanfare music, even the radio will do. Listening to music can take your mind off the drudgery part of doing deep knee bends. And the rhythm will help you find a rhythm for whatever you're doing.

### Join an Athletic Club

Your local sports club can provide more than a pool and a few courts; it can provide a whole ready-made environment where exercise, far from being the side dish, is the main event. Here you can practice your favorite exercise, learn a new one, and take nourishment from an atmosphere consecrated to physical fitness. Most clubs feature both a sauna and steam and whirlpool baths—just the things for relaxing your muscles and shoring up your shipwrecked attitude. A club membership can be on the expensive side, but it is one of the best health insurance policies you could ever take out. Just be sure you go over your contract with the club carefully, so you understand exactly what rights and privileges are yours once you sign up. Many colleges and universities let you have access to their athletic facilities if you enroll in just a single course.

## Sport for Thought

By now, many people have discovered for themselves that meditation is one of the keys to unwinding and thereby to unfolding some extraordinary truths about themselves and their natures (what *they* had always taken for confusion might just turn out to contain a hidden unity!). Meditation is especially beneficial when you practice your aerobic exercise, which is very repetitive. And while you're jogging, try concentrating on your breathing; count your inhalations till you reach the round number ten, then begin all over again. Repetition may not be the spice of life, but it can be awfully relaxing. Think about your breath, where it comes from, where it goes to; clear your mind of all problems, all distractions, all obligations, all entanglements, and in the happy haze that replaces ordered reality, learn to relax.

## Variety

Though I'm faithful to tennis and calisthenics in my fashion, I do like to try new exercises and body movements. There are so many new forms of exercise these days. Weightlifting, for one—a very good way to tone up a flabby body. And women don't have to worry about building unwanted muscles, since they lack the male hormone testosterone. And then there's T'ai Chi, a slow, graceful Chinese calisthenic that greatly improves coordination. And gymnastics, which are especially challenging as they can involve performing stunts. Karate and judo are excellent exercises which can also come in handy. Ice-skating and roller-skating are larky, speedy, and good for your balance and coordination, as are backpacking, fencing, tap-dancing and belly dancing (oooh-la-la, the temperature of the suggested exercises is going up!).

## Find a Friend to Do It With

Man is by nature a companionable animal; he doesn't like to do most things by himself. Exercising with a friend can take the sting out of working out. You may even find that your friend brings out in you the spirit of friendly competition and you push yourself even harder. And with him or her running along beside you, you'll be much less inclined to throw in the towel after the first half mile; under the glare of a little friendly peer pressure, you won't want to lag and shuffle.

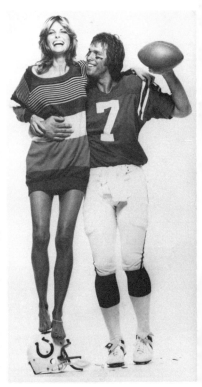

I found Burt Jones of the Baltimore Colts.

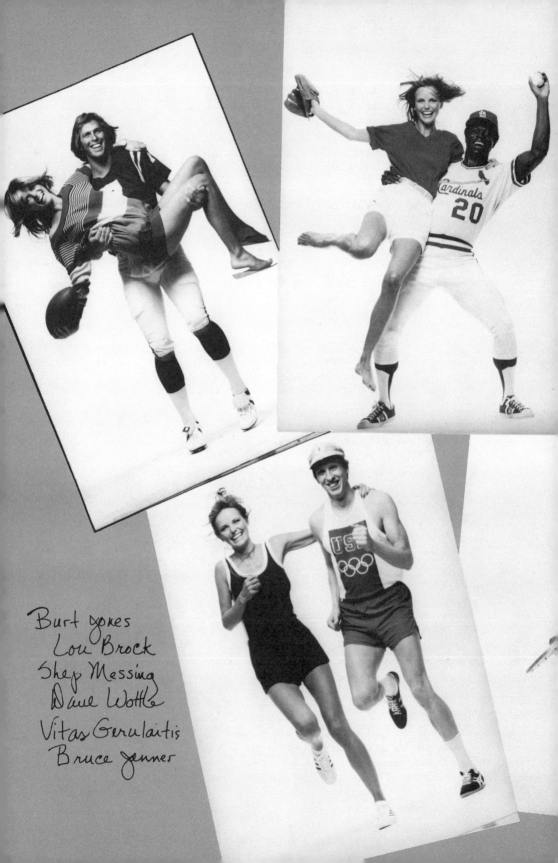

Burt Jones
Lou Brock
Shep Messing
Dave Wottle
Vitas Gerulaitis
Bruce Jenner

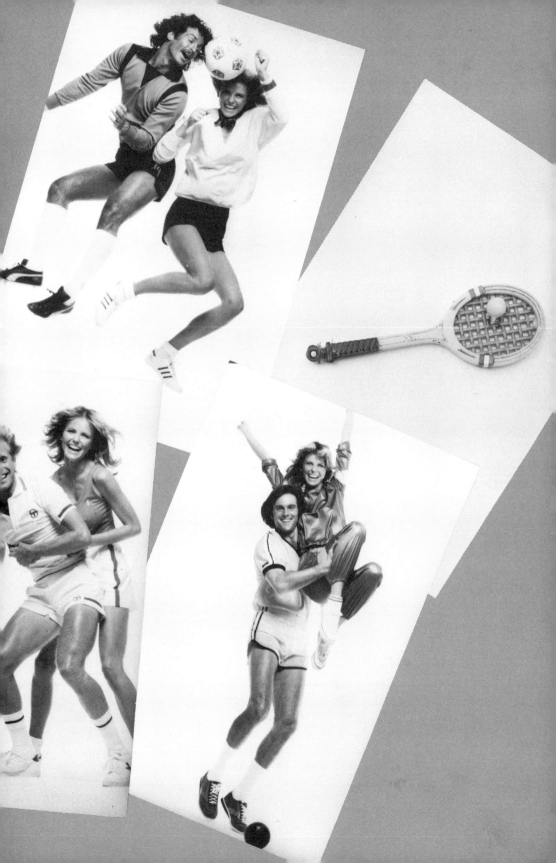

## Professional Help

Any exercise or sport that demands a special physical skill or technique should be embarked upon only with professional instruction. In other words, let the unlimber beware! Errors have a way of compounding—and then perpetuating—themselves. You can injure yourself badly, self-destruct—or simply self-efface. I played tennis off and on for years, loving every heady minute of it. Then one day I decided I just didn't want my game to stay at the same level forever, I wanted to lift myself up into the company of the first-rate. The tactile satisfaction of the game was no longer enough; I had really had it with being mediocre. What I did was take lessons every day for an entire summer. I can't tell you how many times there were when I just couldn't seem to get that serve right, and the quest for the perfect serve was getting me down. But when the frenzy of the lessons had subsided and the strength of my frustrations had grown less, I could see that my technique had improved dramatically. My coach, Bill Regas, was so incredibly patient. At the end of that summer, he wrote me tenderly, in that fierce tennis-hand of his, "I had to sweep a lot of crocodile tears off the court, but I knew that you'd *finally* get it right." Would you call that a backhanded compliment? I would. But at least it wasn't an empty one: He knew I'd never be a Chris Evert but he was pleased that I hadn't settled for mediocrity.

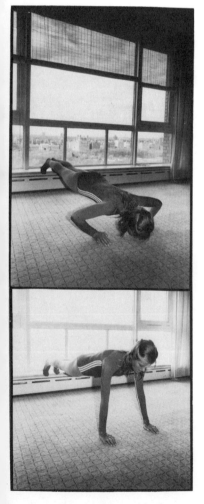

## Hang in There

In order to become good at any sport or exercise, the one thing you have to have is patience. The benefits of exercise are often slow showing up, as they are in some other important areas of your life—career and relationships, for instance. But the day will come when you can measure in all-too-real inches the flesh you've lost around the thighs; when you can clock the number of miles you're able to run; when you can actually see the glow and feel the tingle in your cheeks. One of my friends spent six months doing sit-ups without ever feeling anything more uplifting than pain; but she persevered and now she can do a hundred just like that, and for the first time in her adult life her stomach is perfectly flat. Another friend of mine has been swimming religiously for years, and only recently have her narrow shoulders broadened, her pectoral muscles come into their own, and her posture visibly improved. The moral of these two stories is, of course,

"Stick with it—you're not as hopeless as you think you are." And once you see for yourself what exercise can do for you, you'll forget all about the lazy excuses.

## TIME-SAVING SHAPE-UP OR SHIP-OUT EXERCISES

Despite the best intentions (and who doesn't start out with those?), there are going to be days (and daze) and even weeks when busy people simply cannot find the time to slavishly jog, play squash, or attend exercise class. When I'm traveling, for example, it's impossible for me to adhere to my regular exercise schedule. But instead of completely abandoning my commitment to physical fitness, I concentrate on the parts of my body that I feel need work the most. My arms have this tendency to become too thin when I neglect them. So, no matter how pressed I am for time, every day I do a few minutes of exercises that add tone and muscle to my arms. The area that most women have to work the hardest on is their stomachs, especially if they sit around a lot. A little work on the stomach every day can make an unbelievable difference—and sit-ups you can do anywhere, even in bed!

With the aid of an expert, Tone Vogt, a Norwegian exercise teacher who's kept a lot of the best bodies in Hollywood together, I've designed a time-saving exercise program for people who think they're too busy to bother. These spot exercises are designed to burn fat cells in particular areas of your body; they'll also activate your muscle cells, and build new ones. There are already plenty of exercises for improving the thighs, stomach, buttocks, and arms, so I've gone and chosen only those that will affect more than one part of your body at the same time. The push-ups I recommend primarily for your arms will also strengthen and tone the muscles of your abdomen, buttocks, shoulders, and chest. Better yet, you can do all these exercises in a small space without any equipment at all. When I travel, I just spread a towel on the floor of my hotel room and . . . press on!

In all of the exercises that follow, keep your stomach muscles flat. And remember to breathe in through your nose and out through your mouth, taking care to exhale at the most strenuous part of each exercise. Don't be afraid to let your breath whoosh out. (Just think of it as energy that's helping to activate and relax each and every muscle in your body.) If you hold your

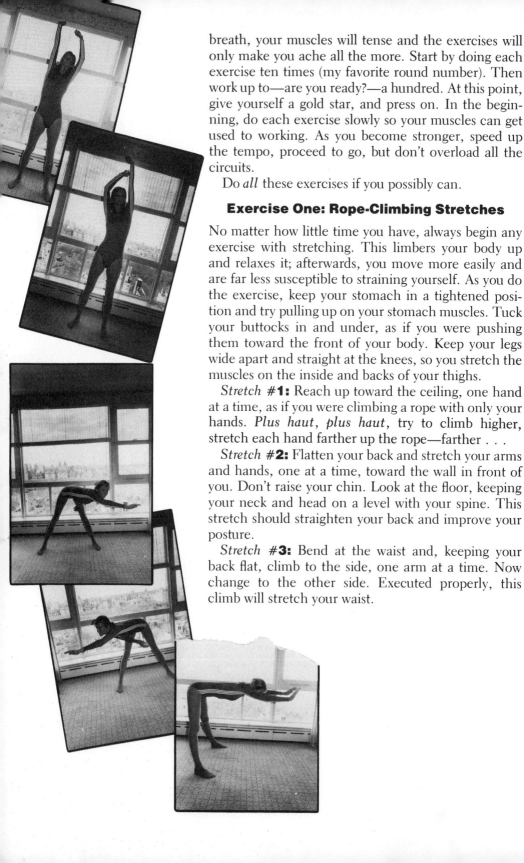

breath, your muscles will tense and the exercises will only make you ache all the more. Start by doing each exercise ten times (my favorite round number). Then work up to—are you ready?—a hundred. At this point, give yourself a gold star, and press on. In the beginning, do each exercise slowly so your muscles can get used to working. As you become stronger, speed up the tempo, proceed to go, but don't overload all the circuits.

Do *all* these exercises if you possibly can.

### Exercise One: Rope-Climbing Stretches

No matter how little time you have, always begin any exercise with stretching. This limbers your body up and relaxes it; afterwards, you move more easily and are far less susceptible to straining yourself. As you do the exercise, keep your stomach in a tightened position and try pulling up on your stomach muscles. Tuck your buttocks in and under, as if you were pushing them toward the front of your body. Keep your legs wide apart and straight at the knees, so you stretch the muscles on the inside and backs of your thighs.

*Stretch #1:* Reach up toward the ceiling, one hand at a time, as if you were climbing a rope with only your hands. *Plus haut, plus haut,* try to climb higher, stretch each hand farther up the rope—farther . . .

*Stretch #2:* Flatten your back and stretch your arms and hands, one at a time, toward the wall in front of you. Don't raise your chin. Look at the floor, keeping your neck and head on a level with your spine. This stretch should straighten your back and improve your posture.

*Stretch #3:* Bend at the waist and, keeping your back flat, climb to the side, one arm at a time. Now change to the other side. Executed properly, this climb will stretch your waist.

## Exercise Two: Inner Thigh Bounces

Because few of us use our inner thigh muscles in our everyday activities, they get flabby and sag more rapidly than most other parts of our body. I've invented a simple and very effective exercise to activate the inner thigh muscles: the "bounce." Place your legs as wide apart as you can without losing your balance. Turn your toes out. Now, keeping your buttocks tucked under and your stomach tight, bend your knees as much as you can and bounce up and down without ever straightening your knees. If you're doing it right, you should be able to feel your inner thigh muscles tighten. Bounce for at least a minute.

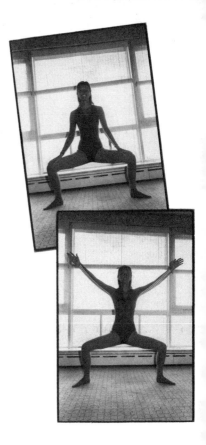

*Arm Bounces.* Proceed as in the inner thigh bounce, except this time raise your arms to shoulder length. Your palms should be facing the wall in front of you and your hands and fingers should be stretched. Make ten big circles forward with your arms, then ten backward. Then make ten *small* circles forward *and* backward. Keep your fingers stretched, elbows locked, and move your arms and shoulder. What you're doing is firming up the tricep muscles that keep the underside of your upper arms smooth and taut. Combining the two exercises is a real time-saver.

## Exercise Three: C.T.'s Friendly Feminine Push-up

Most women don't have enough strength in their arms and shoulders to do push-ups, an old standby if there ever was one for firming and toning arms and shoulders. I've tailored the following exercise especially to women.

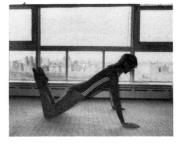

Lie on your stomach. Bend your knees and cross your ankles. Place your hands on the floor right next to your shoulders. Your knees should be resting on the carpet. Raise the upper part of your body with your arms. Now lower your body back down till it's almost touching the floor. Raise it up again using your arms. (Don't konk out between push-ups.) Keep your buttocks and stomach tight. The top of your body should be all in a straight line. It's hard work but well worth it —this exercise will firm up not only your buttocks and stomach, but also the muscles in your arms, shoulders, and chest. Remember to exhale when you raise your body, and inhale when you lower it.

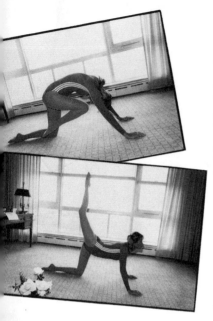

### Exercise Four: The Cat Stretch (Without Claws)

This exercise will stretch the muscles in your abdomen and neck as well as tone your buttocks, the backs of your legs, and that problem area under your chin. Get down on all fours. Come on, really crouch. Your elbows should be straight, your hands under your shoulders, and your knees six to eight inches apart. Now bring one knee up to your forehead, then stretch the leg through and back, lifting it as high as you can make it go and keeping that knee really straight. Good, that's it. Exhale as you lift your leg, and lift your chin, too, so that you're looking up at the ceiling. When you kick your leg up, you're stretching the muscles in your abdomen, working the area under your buttocks, and firming the buttocks themselves, which are so damn hard to firm. If you have a bad back, don't lift your leg up, just stretch it back toward the wall. Repeat—guess how many times on each side? Ten!

### Exercise Five: The Dreaded Hydrant

Unlike most of the other exercises I do, this one activates a part of the body that seldom even moves. It's an exercise guaranteed to trim and tone the fat that invariably, furtively, gathers on the outside of women's thighs and hangs on for dear life even after you've vigorously dieted. It firms the area just *beneath* the buttocks as well.

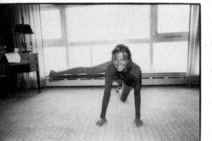

Get ready, get set . . . Get down on your hands and knees the way you just did in the cat exercise. Put your right leg out to the side and lift it as high as you can. Keep your knee straight and your foot flexed, so you stretch the hamstring muscle on the back of your thigh. Now raise and lower your leg ten times—keeping it straight. Now make ten circles forward with your leg and ten backward. If it hurts, well, it *should* hurt (doesn't everything good hurt a little?). It should hurt right around where all that fat is. Now do the same thing with the left leg. The same number of times. Keep your whole body straight; don't lean away from the extended leg. It's better to lower the leg a little than to lean and go easy on yourself.

### Exercise Six: The Half Sit-up

"Ah," you're thinking, "the sit-up—an old, old friend." This version of it, however, won't be all that familiar to you. If it's your lower abdomen you want to tone and strengthen, lie on your back, lift your legs straight up and cross them at the ankles. Then clasp your hands behind your head so your elbows are at right angles to your body. Now, keeping your elbows back and parallel to the floor, lift the upper part of your body toward your knees. Exhale as you come up, inhale as you go back down. You'll probably get your chin only as far as your chest, but even so you'll feel the muscles working in your lower abdomen. If it's the upper part of your abdomen, near the waist, that needs work, bend your elbows toward your knees as you raise the upper part of your body.

### Exercise Seven: Lifting Your Legs

This one is hard on the lower back, but give it a chance, it's an excellent stomach flattener. Rest your elbows on the floor, legs straight, lock your knees, and flex your feet to stretch your hamstrings. Raise your legs up and let them down without allowing them to touch the floor. If you can't lift both legs at the same time, scissor them or lift them one at a time, alternating them—but, again, don't let them touch the floor for even a second. Practice control; don't throw them up and down.

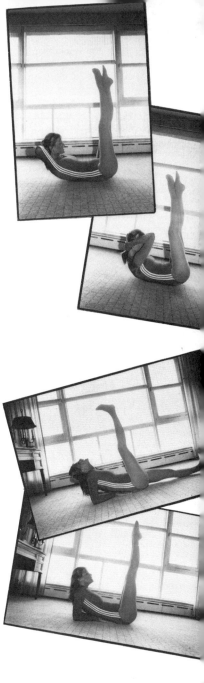

## RELAXATION EXERCISES OR PARDON MY OXYMORON

Relaxation is not the least important part of exercise. The following exercises will all relax your back and neck.

### Relaxation Exercise #1: The Plow

The plow (you're probably imagining the snow crunching under it) is much more beatific than it sounds. What it is is a well-known hatha-yoga exercise, unsurpassable for relaxing and stretching your back and neck muscles. Lie on your back with your hands resting beside your thighs, palms down. Lift your legs slowly (if you've put on snowboots to do The Plow, kick them off), keep them straight, and bring them over your head till your toes touch the floor. Keep your knees straight and together now. Press your chin into your chest. Try to make your breath rush into the parts of your back that feel tense and achy. Hold this position for as long as you humanly can; don't worry, it will get more comfortable as the tension empties out of your back. You get a feeling that's hard to explain.

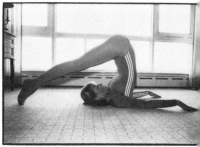

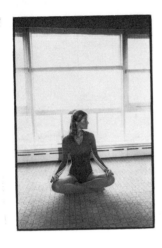

### Relaxation Exercise #2: Head and Spine Stretches

Sit in a cross-legged position. Keep erect (a good way to do this is to imagine that there's an invisible string pulling your head up toward the ceiling). Pull up on your stomach and chest muscles. Now stretch your left ear down toward your shoulder, then your right ear. Then, moving slowly, turn your head to the back and push your chin toward your left shoulder. Do the same now on the right side. Strain to see the wall behind you, and strain hard, because this is what helps prevent a double chin. Now make full circles with your head—to the right, to the back, to the left, and *down*, in a clockwise, then counterclockwise rotation.

### Relaxation Exercise #3: Hanging Down

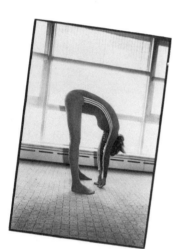

Stand with your legs straight and apart, then let your head drop toward your feet as low as you can go. Think of the upper part of your body as a dead weight: you're an old rag doll, your arms dangle, your head and neck loll. Then roll yourself up slowly to a standing position. This is a good thing to do between exercises, when you're feeling all tuckered out.

## C.T.'S MINUTE-TO-MINUTE GUIDE TO KEEPING YOUR SHAPE

Every woman needs to set part of her week aside for vigorous exercise sessions. I also happen to be a great believer in informal exercises you can do throughout the day. These "invisible" exercises involve substituting movement for non-movement at every opportunity, using more muscles to do your ordinary activities, and doing the special isometric "mini" exercises that you can do almost anywhere. These "invisible" exercises can make the difference, the not "invisible," in fact the very, very visible—difference—in your shape.

### Walk Briskly

Everybody has to walk. But there's more than one way to do it, that's for sure. You can just shuffle along, barely moving your body, or you can walk exuberantly, exercising as many muscles as possible. When I walk, I keep my shoulders up and back, and pull up on my stomach muscles. As I take each step, I stretch and tighten the backs of my legs. I try to keep up a good pace. All this makes walking a real pleasure. More importantly, it improves my muscle tone and my cardiovascular system. A test conducted by the University of California at Irvine showed that fat women lose approximately twenty-two pounds during their diet programs simply by walking more than half an hour each day. Do yourself a big favor: try it my way—walking instead of riding whenever possible. Prove to yourself that you retain the power of locomotion.

## Climb Those Stairs

I'm lucky to live in a two-story house, because climbing stairs does wonders for legs, buttocks, and abdominal muscles. Whenever I can avoid taking an elevator, I do. And when I climb, I pull up on my stomach muscles and take the stairs as quickly as I can. And as for escalators, don't just stand there, nodding or dozing—walk up them!

## Use That Beach

The beach is nature's health club and if you're smart, you'll treat it as such. Most people just spread their blankets on the sand, smear themselves with suntan oil, and lie there recklessly exposing their skin to the sun. When I'm at the beach, I run. Running on sand is better for calf muscles and feet than running on dirt or cement. I jog through the surf, lifting my feet high. And back on the beach, I dig my toes deep into the sand to stretch and strengthen my feet. The beach is also a great place for playing frisbee, volleyball, or football. And, in case somebody hasn't noticed it yet, it's not a bad place for swimming.

## See C.T. Run

If I'm working out-of-doors and the changing room is a ways away, I jog there. Even when I don't jog regularly, I do try an occasional sprint. (People look at me kind of funny, as if I must be late to something.) Try running to get your newspaper in the morning, run to catch the bus, try outrunning your dog (if he's fifteen and he overtakes you, you've learned a hard truth). Then, if you're ever being chased by a rampaging herd of elephants, you'll be able to run . . . for your life!

## Do!

Dance after dinner—it'll help you work off a big meal. Bicycle. Bowl. Play Ping-Pong. Roller-skate. These are all energetic alternatives to an evening spent at home cautiously lashed to your chair.

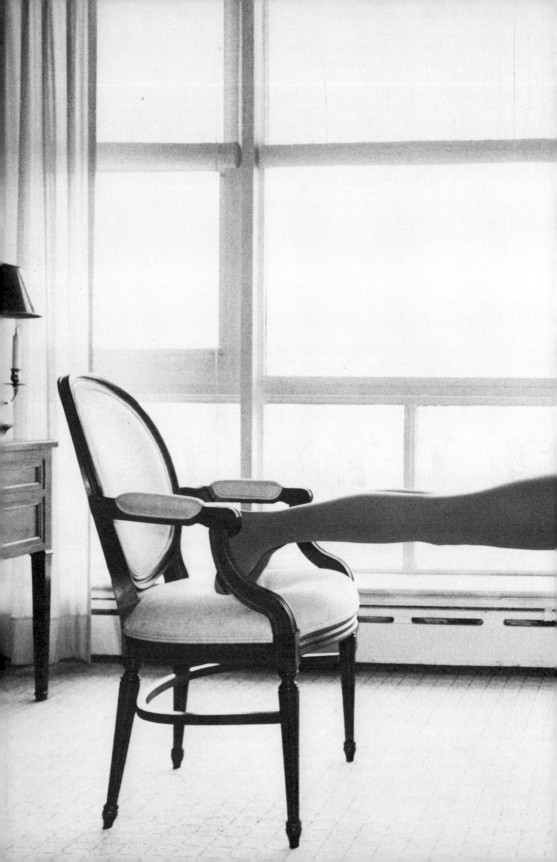

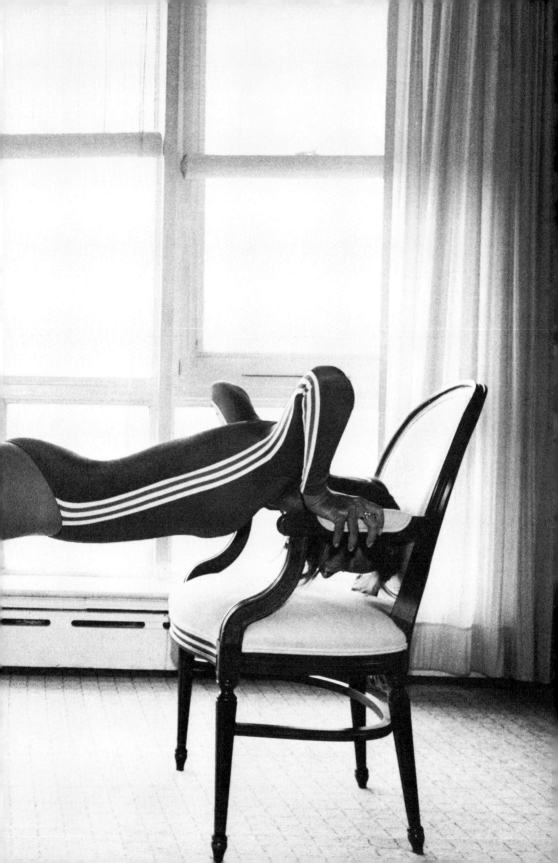

The simple isometric exercises that follow you can do in an office, an uncrowded elevator, or at home. They take almost no time at all. Best of all, you don't even have to change clothes.

### Stomach Press

Breathe out all the air in your lungs, then press your stomach with your palms, keeping your elbows at right angles to your body. Continue to breathe deeply, inhaling through your nose and exhaling through your mouth. But keep pressing your stomach as hard as you can with both hands. You want to firm your stomach as well as your upper arms, don't you?

### Wall Push

Fold your arms in front of you at chest level, grasping each forearm with the opposite hand. Now push against both arms simultaneously with short, jerking motions. Ahh! This exercise will tone both the muscles that support your breasts and those in your upper arms.

### Weighting By the Phone

Stand at least an arm's length away from a wall with your feet a few inches apart. Now place your palms on the wall. Lean right into the wall so your elbows bend, then push yourself away. Don't lift your heels. This modified, easy-to-do version of the push-ups you do on the floor will keep your arms and wrists in shape.

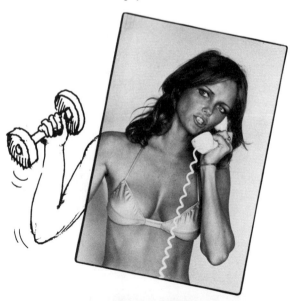

128

### Pick-ups/Pick-me-ups/
### Pick-me-up-off-the-floor-oops

Are your lower back and the hamstring muscles in the backs of your legs so stiff you can't even touch your toes? Then try keeping your legs and knees straight and bending from the waist whenever you have to pick something up from the floor. That way, you're doing what amounts to a toe touch every time you pick up a fallen pencil or something. As hard as I tried, I couldn't touch my toes till I made this exercise part of my everyday life. You shouldn't try to pick up a two-hundred-pound object this way, though—you don't want to injure your back.

### Kick up the Door

This is my invention, a version of a ballet exercise called the *grand battement* that's great for thighs and abdomens. Hold both sides of a door jamb with your hands and kick up a storm, ten times with each leg; then kick to the back ten times. The secret is to pull up on your stomach muscles and keep your posture erect while you kick as high as you can (don't bend to meet your leg as it rises).

### Stomach Press

Breathe out all the air in your lungs, then press your stomach with your palms, keeping your elbows at right angles to your body. Continue to breathe deeply, inhaling through your nose and exhaling through your mouth. But keep pressing your stomach as hard as you can with both hands. You want to firm your stomach as well as your upper arms, don't you?

### Arm Push

Fold your arms in front of you at chest level, grasping each forearm with the opposite hand. Now push against both arms simultaneously with short, jerking motions. Ahh! This exercise will tone both the muscles that support your breasts and those in your upper arms.

### Stretch and Sigh

When I'm feeling restless or lethargic from working really hard, I get up and stretch. When I'm tense, I suck in all the air I can get and then let it all out in a huge, noisy, earthshaking sigh. This habit, which by now is involuntary with me, has produced some weird and worried looks on the faces of those around me, but my accumulated tension sure disappears—and so do some of the weirdos nearby.

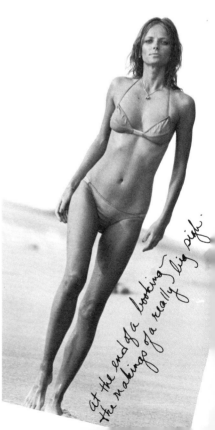

*at the end of a booking, the makings of a really big sigh*

## Overdoing It

It *is* possible to exercise too much. A couple of summers ago when I was playing tennis regularly and also taking three weekly calisthenic classes, I found I was listless most of the time, and ready to fall into sleep (as if into an open grave) right after an early dinner. My entire system was protesting that it had had too much! If you overswim, overjog, or otherwise overdo, your body will let you know it sooner or later, one way or another. So learn to listen to it. Don't overdo—over-don't.

## Giving up too Soon

To get the most out of exercise you have to push yourself a bit beyond the comfortable limit. The best time to do three extra sit-ups or push-ups is at exactly the point when the muscles you're using begin to ache—it's those few extra motions that do the trick. When you're doing an aerobic exercise such as jogging, it's crucial that you go a bit longer and further than you ever thought you could. The line between overdoing it and getting enough is a very thin one. Don't worry about ordinary muscle soreness; treat yourself to a good massage, or a colossal bath with Epsom salts. And don't wait till the soreness has disappeared completely before going back to the exercise. More exercise will, in fact, ease the pain. So keep pushing yourself. It won't kill you; it will do you a lot of good (said she, puffing and panting).

## Overeating Before or After Exercising

Don't eat right before you exercise unless you want to feel sick to your stomach. Eat no less than two hours before calisthenics and three hours before a competitive event.

I've known so many people who've used their half-hour exercise session to justify eating a pint of ice cream later on. "I burned up so many calories," they all say, "I can afford to give myself a little treat. In fact," they escalate, "I positively owe it to myself." What's so surprising is how surprised they always are to see the pounds pile up. If you're going to play *that* game, bring a calculator along—I'm not kidding—so that after you've jogged for twenty minutes, you know it's 300 calories you've burned up and not the eight million contained in a pint of ice cream. Fair is fair—and fun is fun (and fun is over).

## Crash-Dieting While Exercising

A crash diet and a rigorous exercise regimen combined can throw your whole system out of sync. So, if you are dieting *and* exercising at the same time, make sure that you're eating a varied, nutritious 1200 calories a day. You see, when you exercise, muscle mass increases as fat decreases, so that you may weigh the same even though you look much thinner. If this is the case, only your tape measure will know for sure.

## Kid Yourself Not: No-Exercise Exercising

Some people kid themselves that they're exercising when what they're doing is more like play. Machines that jiggle your flesh around are no substitute for exercise, for the simple reason they don't make demands on your muscles. A good game of golf may relax you but, as it involves hardly any muscle activity at all, it does not qualify as a fitness exercise. Walking is naturally far better for you than riding in a car, but walking alone will not keep you in shape. Any exercise that involves a lot of stops and starts and that isn't done strenuously won't give you real and lasting benefits, either. Floating on your back in a lake under an amazing summer sky, for instance, is no more *swimming* than a big icicle is a bed of flowers!

## Not Concentrating

When you exercise, you should be thinking of nothing else but how that exercise feels and what it is doing to your body. I've seen women in exercise classes casually throw their arms and legs around while they laugh and yak and live it up. Well, let's see how much good *that* does them! By concentrating, you will very likely find the one way to do each exercise which makes *your* muscles work harder. You become aware of each part of your body, of how the muscles there connect to muscles elsewhere. If you concentrate on your exercise, you become better at it more quickly and enjoy it more. When you do your calisthenics, don't just watch yourself in the mirror (tempting as that might be); instead, think about how the exercises feel. Much of what happens to you is in the brain, after all—so use it!

## Crossing Your Legs

Fine, go right ahead, if you want to cut off the circulation in your thighs. Remember, "cellulite" loves a vacuum.

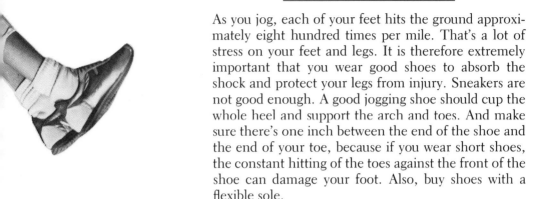

## FOOTGEAR FOR RUNNING

As you jog, each of your feet hits the ground approximately eight hundred times per mile. That's a lot of stress on your feet and legs. It is therefore extremely important that you wear good shoes to absorb the shock and protect your legs from injury. Sneakers are not good enough. A good jogging shoe should cup the whole heel and support the arch and toes. And make sure there's one inch between the end of the shoe and the end of your toe, because if you wear short shoes, the constant hitting of the toes against the front of the shoe can damage your foot. Also, buy shoes with a flexible sole.

## THE BODY PRESENTABLE
## VS. THE BODY IMPOSSIBLE

When you exercise, aspire to a realistic version of your present body. No amount of exercise can change your basic proportions or transform your body type from, let's say, soft and round to thin and angular, since exercise is a form neither of magic nor of sorcery. Certain body types, such as those that are heavy from the waist down and slim on top, can be improved, and that's all. What you should look for exercise to do is make the body you already have just as fit and attractive as it was biologically "programmed" to be. And to do that, we have to find out our own rhythm and make our own breakthroughs.

In A *Separate Peace*, one of the most moving books I read in high school, Finny, a fifteen-year-old injured former athlete, coaches his prep-school friend Gene to run the course that he himself can no longer run: "four times around an oval walk which circled the Headmaster's home, a large rambling, doubtfully Colonial white mansion." Here is Gene's account:

> . . . *After making two circuits of the walk every trace of energy was as usual completely used up, and as I drove myself on all my scattered aches found their usual way to a profound seat of pain in my side. My lungs as usual were fed up with all this work, and from now on would only go rackingly through the motions. My knees were boneless again, ready any minute to let my lower legs telescope up into the thighs. My head felt as though different sections of the cranium were grinding into each other.*

Then, for no reason at all, I felt magnificent. It was as though my body until that instant had simply been lazy, as though the aches and exhaustion were all imagined, created from nothing in order to keep me from truly exerting myself. Now my body seemed at last to say, "Well, if you must have it, here!" and an accession of strength came flooding through me. Buoyed up, I forgot my usual feeling of routine self-pity when working out, I lost myself, oppressed mind along with aching body; all entanglements were shed, I broke into the clear.

After the fourth circuit, like sitting in a chair, I pulled up in front of Phineas.

"You're not even winded," he said.

"I know."

"You found your rhythm, didn't you, that third time around. Just as you came into that straight part there."

"Yes, right there."

"You've been pretty lazy all along, haven't you?"

"Yes, I guess I have been."

"You didn't even know anything about yourself."

"I don't guess I did, in a way."

"Well," he gathered the sheepskin collar around his throat, "now you know. . . ."

Yes. As the good book says, so now you know.

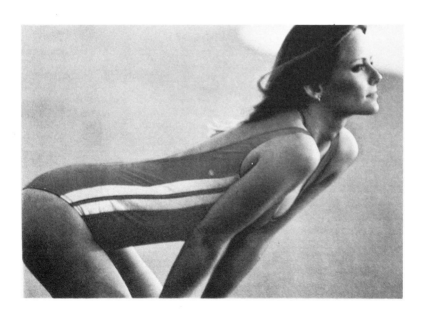

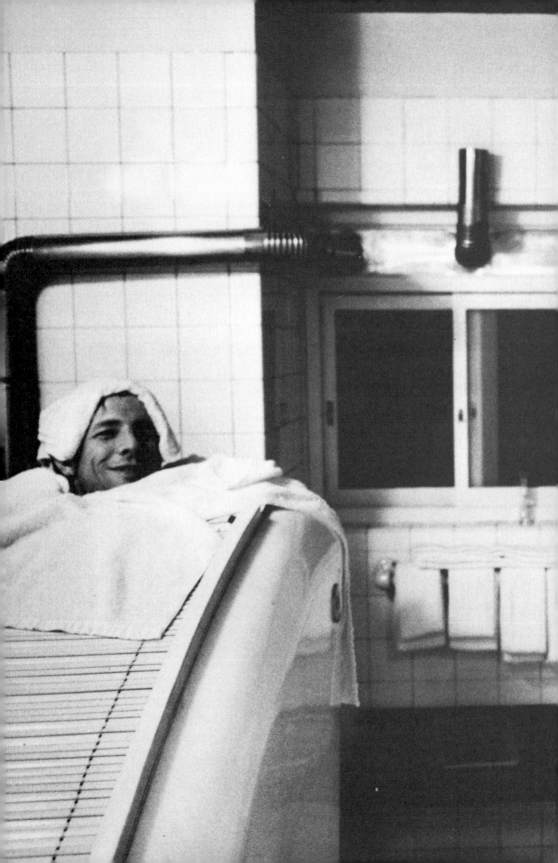

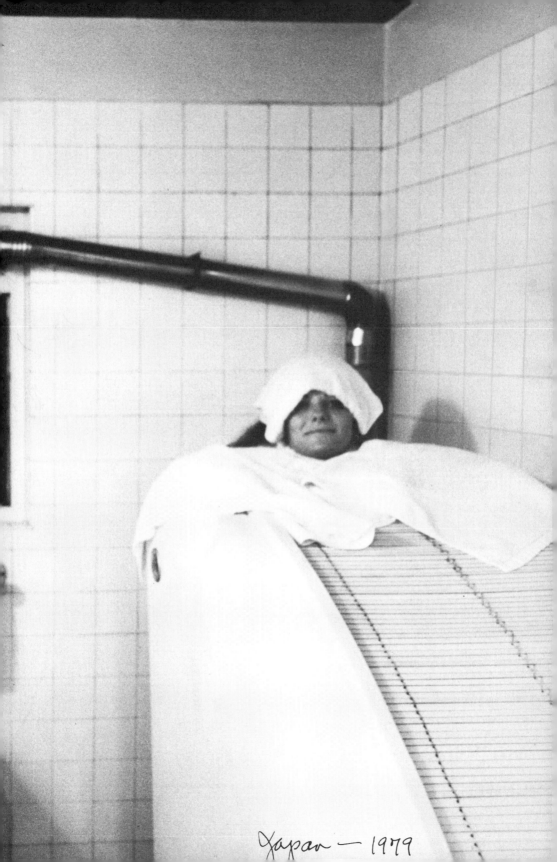

Japan — 1979

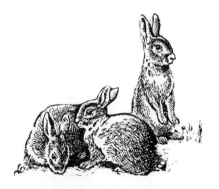

# 5

## Hair Today, Hair Tomorrow: Using Your Head

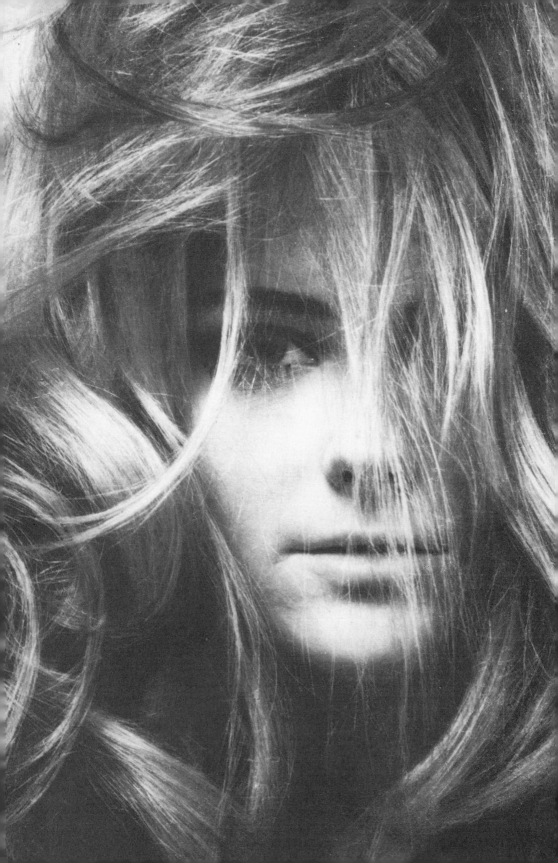

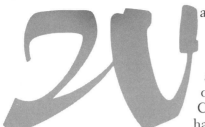ay back in the eleventh century, Leofric, Earl of Mercia, imposed a burdensome tax on the people of Coventry. And what has this got to do with hair? you're thinking. Well, wait and see. When his wife importuned him to remit the tax, he jestingly promised to do so if she would ride naked through the streets of the town at noonday. She took him at his word, directed the people to keep within doors and close their shutters, and complied with his condition. (Peeping Tom, who looked out, was struck blind.) Her act was not quite so daring as it might have been, because she knew that her entire naked front and back would be covered by her fabulous long blond hair. The lady's name, of course, was Godiva, and that town owes a whole lot to the fact that she had hair to spare, hair that simply would not quit.

And who has not been moved by O. Henry's great short story, "The Gift of the Magi"? The two young people are married and starving, and Christmas is coming up. The woman goes and sells the only possession she has, her extraordinarily long chestnut hair, in order to buy her husband a gold watch chain for his prized family watch, but meanwhile—unbeknownst to her—he has sold the watch in order to buy her combs for her glorious hair.

Hair was the O. Henry heroine's most treasured possession, and it is also one of yours. Shining, healthy hair, attractively cut and styled, is the greatest pleasure, the most tactile satisfaction. It provides a frame for your face, and unlike your figure and your skin, is easy to utterly transform. Within a few hours your hair can have a vivid new coloring, a different texture, or a dramatic new style (as the Clairesse ad says, "Go Glamorous").

But changing your hair color or style takes not only thought but knowledge. In a novel I just read, one of the characters has red hair, and her husband's boss says to him threateningly, "Your wife is a good woman, I'm sure. But that hair . . . there ought to be some way to tone it down." The poor woman probably didn't know how.

Is your hair doing the most it can for you? And are you doing all you can for it? Here are some questions for you to stub your big toe against.

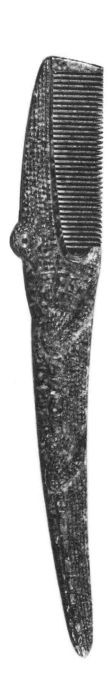

■ *Have you had the same hairstyle for years?*

■ *Do you usually wind up regretting having had your hair cut, or changing the color or style, because the results are not what you'd hoped for?*

■ *If you hair is colored, do you insist on the colors being uniform throughout?*

■ *Do you feel that in order for your hair to look attractive, you have to set it?*

■ *Do you think it's a good idea to give your hair a hundred brushstrokes every day?*

■ *If, after a haircut, you part your hair on either side or in the middle, does it fall evenly and frame your face appealingly?*

■ *Do you wash your hair every day?*

■ *Does your hair become limp and separate into strands shortly after you wash it?*

■ *Do you use deep conditioning treatments for the split ends?*

■ *Do you always have your permanent done by a professional?*

Your answer to the first five questions should be an emphatic "no!"

In this chapter I hope to help you find an exciting hairstyle that reflects the person you are *now*, not someone you were—or think you were—years ago. If you want to look like the ideal picture of yourself, take care that you don't wind up looking like a picture frame out of which the picture has dropped.

Plan your hairstyle realistically, with *your* face and *your* hair type and *your* everyday activities in mind. And don't just hand over the entire responsibility to your stylist—you're going to have to learn to work with him. He'll know how not to make you a slave to your hair; on the contrary, he'll see to it that your hair is easy to care for and that it looks good whether you set it or not. And, yes, Virginia, a good haircut will fall into place no matter where you part it.

There are no hard-and-fast rules for how often you should brush your hair or even wash it. Frequent shampooing won't necessarily harm your hair, as many people believe. And as you will see, it's possible to stop ends from splitting with conditioners. As for hair that's artificially colored, it should contain the same highlights and varied shades as natural hair color does, or it will look lifeless.

## WHAT YOUR HAIR HAS TO SAY ABOUT YOU

A woman's hairstyle makes a statement not only about how she sees herself but about how she wants to be seen by others, who she wants them to take her for. Whether your hairstyle is drab and pedestrian, free and flowing, a complete mad raucous mass of wild curls that practically swallows everyone and everything in its path, or so elaborate and baroque that it all but bumps against the ceiling, the truth about how you see yourself will out. If a hairstyle isn't flattering to your face, it won't feel all that comfortable and won't reflect what I hesitate to call "the real you" (which may be somebody you don't even know yet, or have merely a nodding acquaintance with).

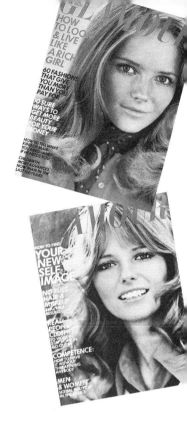

When I'm modeling I usually rebel if the stylist tries to overload my hair with flamboyant flips, a pageboy, you name it. I feel totally unconnected to them (and to myself when I'm wearing them). I always encourage the stylist to fluff out my hair so it looks natural and unfettered, and I discourage him from spraying and teasing. I like my hair to look about the same in a photograph as it does in real life, because publicly and privately, I try to stay pretty much the same person. (It's a battle, I can tell you.)

A hairstyle should take into consideration the shape of your face and the type of hair you have, but there's more than one attractive style for every woman. I've often changed hairstyles. And in the process I've noticed that outer changes really do mirror inner ones, so that a hairstyle that's left over from some part of your past is going to look and feel like the most unwieldy anachronism.

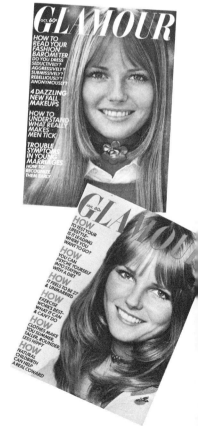

I'm always having my hair layered, then letting the layers grow out, or getting a permanent for more body and pizzazz, or highlighting my hair with streaks of color. Like most people, I don't have endless blocks of time to spend on my grooming, so I strive to make my hair look attractive without my having to resort to curling irons, curlers, and a lot of other time-consum-

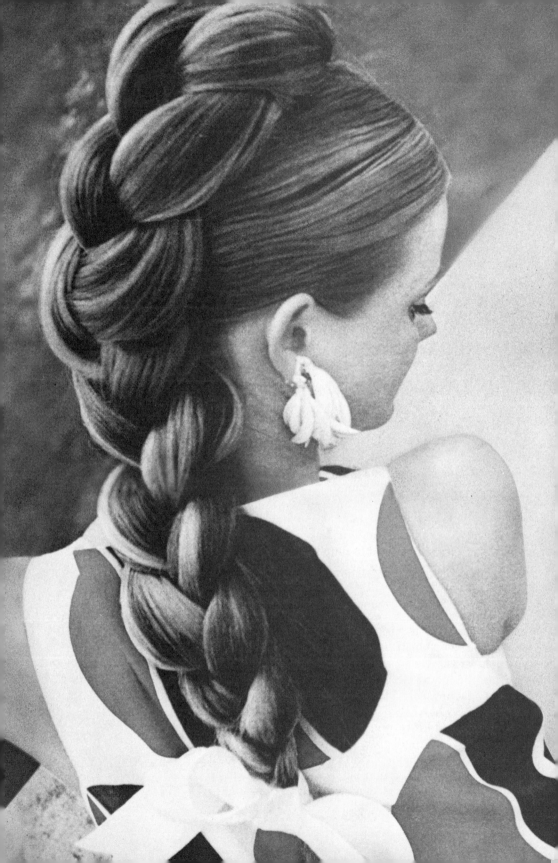

ing paraphernalia. All I want to have to do is wash it, fluff it, and let it dry—nothing much more esoteric than that, if you please. Of course, for special occasions, I actually enjoy taking the extra time out to curl my hair and maybe even stud it with sparkling combs and barrettes so it'll look . . . well, spectacular!

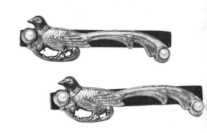

## CHOOSING THE RIGHT STYLE

Any hairstylist worth his blow-dryer will take care to emphasize your best features. And so should you. If you have beautiful big eyes, a firm chin line, or sculpted cheekbones, you should choose a hairstyle that makes the most of these assets. Hair pulled back and away from the upper half of your face, for example, will display your eyes and cheekbones to their best advantage. Hair scraped back into a sophisticated chignon, however, may not be very becoming to a long chin, or to a nose that's not as small or well-shaped as you might wish it were. But just a few wisps of bangs can camouflage a wide forehead, and a long chin or jawline can be softened by long hair fluffed and curled on either side of your face. The most important thing to bear in mind is that there are no stiff rules governing the correspondence between a woman's hairstyle and her face. Some of the most attractive styles I've seen on friends are the very ones that, if they'd gone by the book, they would never in a million years have dared to experiment with. (One of my friends, who has a large, slightly crooked nose, looks great with her hair pulled severely back off her face and into a bun on top of her head.) Hairstyles don't exist by themselves, their surroundings are important, to say the least—and their surroundings are none other than *your face*. Every style that works well with a face does so in a mysterious, often totally unpredictable way.

Your body figures into all of this, too. Your hairstyle must balance out the proportions of the body, which is no alien zone as far as hair goes. A very short woman may find that her long straight hair literally buries her underneath it. I have a long, thin body, and a very short cut would be a big mistake on me. Very full, bushy hair on a large woman won't exactly give a slimming illusion—on the contrary: it will make her look hopelessly bulky, as if she could fill the whole back of a taxicab all by herself.

The style you choose should depend not only on the shape of your body and face but on the quality of your

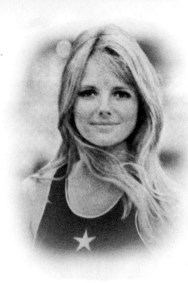

hair as well. Although today chemical processes can alter hair texture, you should never depend on them wholly to maintain your style. If the style you're after necessitates that you drastically change the natural texture, flow, and direction of your hair, and that you constantly set and/or blow-dry it, forget it, it isn't worth it, it won't change your life anyway. Choose a style that's easy to maintain—not some impossible dream from a fashion magazine.

## GROWING LONG HAIR

A lot of women truly believe that if they have the patience and hold out, their hair will eventually grow to a length to rival Rapunzel's or our old (eleventh century!) friend Lady Godiva's. But, growth is based not on a wishbone but on a genetic program that allows hair to achieve a certain predetermined length only. According to the *AMA Book of Skin and Hair Care*, hair grows at the rate of about half an inch a month, then takes a little rest. During this siesta, the hairs that have reached their maximum length are shed slowly, and new hair begins growing to replace them. Don't get too frustrated if your hair breaks and splits at the ends. You may just be genetically "programmed" to a relatively short hair-growing span, in which case you're far better off accepting the inevitable and sticking to a shorter, easy-to-maintain style. Salon experts advise women who want long hair to have a quarter of an inch trimmed off the ends every two months to insure sleek, healthy looking hair that will fall smoothly into place.

## TRYING NEW STYLES OUT

You should remember, when you up and change hairstyles, that it's going to stay that way for a while. Changing your image, your special imprint, is always a lottery. Careful thought and a bit of experimentation before you take the big plunge will help you make a choice that you know you—and yours—can live with. Never simply surrender yourself to a stylist, because when it's all over you may look into the mirror only to find that, suddenly shorn, the top of your noggin resembles nothing so much as a little guinea pig.

Choose your new hairstyle realistically—bearing in mind not only your face, figure, and hair type, but also your personality—and the amount of time you can afford to spend on maintenance. Fashion magazines

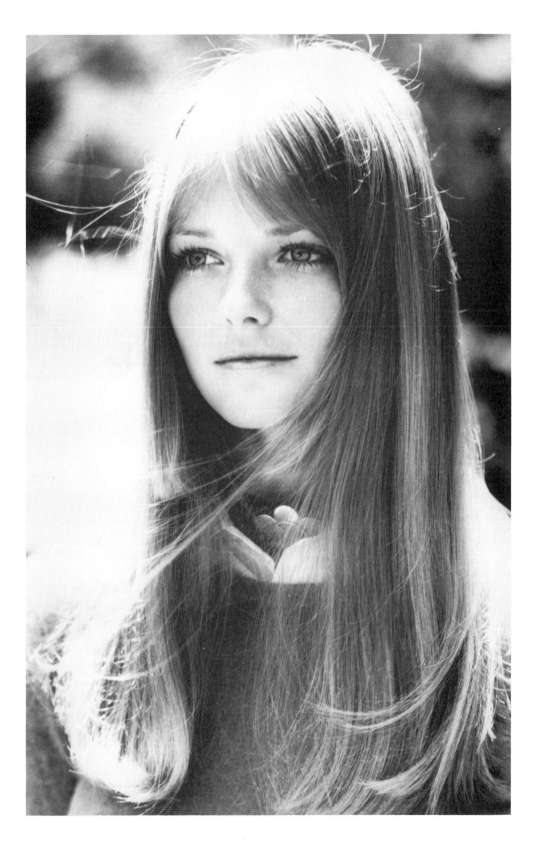

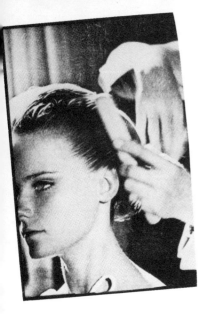

feature fabulous hair styles, concocted by the most inventive stylists. It's all right to be influenced by them, but try not to just copy. Study the type of hair shown in the picture and look carefully at the shape of the model's face. Does it bear more than a passing resemblance to your own hair type and the shape of your own face? Don't go with a style merely because it looks glamorous on someone else! Truth to tell, *you* might be ill-fitted to carry it off.

Wigs and falls can give you some potent clues as to how you're going to look in hair of various lengths and colors. If you're really nervous about changing styles, give a thought to altering the length or color of your hair by degrees. A total change, complete with cut, perm, and new color, may be too extreme for comfort. Consider your nervous system!

## CHOOSING A STYLIST

A good stylist will help you decide on a new hairdo or tell you why the one *you* want isn't quite the right one. Unfortunately, not all stylists are equally talented and well-trained. Creating beautiful hair is an art, requiring study, experience, and skill. Some stylists are at their best with certain types of hair; some are better with people than they are with hair—a salon can be a pretty weird place, a hothouse, a tropical aviary. Finding the best stylist requires some real detective work. Don't make the mistake of thinking that anyone who works in a beauty salon, even a celebrated one, is equipped to cut, color, or perm your one and only head of hair!

If you live in or near a large city, the stars of the hairstyling firmament will be available to you. The personnel in the large, better-known salons are for the most part well trained in modern techniques. If you live in a small town, however, there may not be a single salon equipped to give you a top-quality job. Your hair is so vital to your overall appearance that just this once you should indulge yourself in the luxury of getting the best. If none of the stylists in your immediate area live up to your expectations, drive to the nearest city where top professionals *are* available.

In general, when it comes to hair stylists you get what you pay for. Although it is still possible to get a good haircut for a modest price, the best stylists do command top dollars.

If you have to travel to get a good cut, make sure the

**146** *A day with Kenneth*

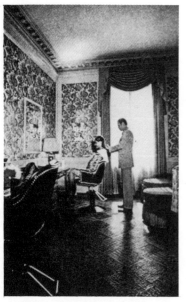

stylist understands that you won't be able to come in very often for trims, and that the style he gives you must grow out gracefully. Once you have a good basic cut, your local stylist may be able to trim it for you himself.

The best way to discover the top stylist in your area is, believe it or not, by observing other women's hair. When you see a winner, don't be embarrassed to ask her for the name of the salon she uses. She'll appreciate the compliment and be happy to tell you. If you are still nervous about taking the inexorable step, just poke your head into the salon and take a quick look around. If you don't like what you see, don't make an appointment—it's as simple as that.

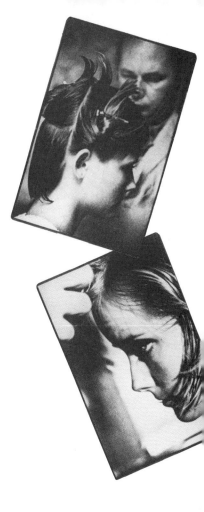

## HOW TO WORK WITH YOUR STYLIST

Once you have a style in mind and a stylist in hand, make the most of him or her. Hairstylists are artists, and more often than not they have the so-called "artistic temperament." Often the spectacular "new you" they long to create is a you fashioned according to their ideas and inspirations. Years ago one stylist insisted I would look glorious if only I would allow him to tint my hair with henna. He was very persuasive, I must say—to the point where I was projecting how much fun it was going to be to have red hair for a change. Luckily, I had a friend who warned me that I wasn't going to want to confront this color every waking hour for the next six months. Remember, a stylist may have the most original and ingenious ideas for your hair, but *he* doesn't have to live with his brilliant creation—*you do*. Yes, of course, listen to his advice, benefit from his training and experience: but don't be afraid to speak up—and not necessarily in a small voice, either.

When you go to a stylist for the first time, make an effort to get your personality across to him. Also, describe the hairstyle you have in mind in very clear terms. Don't say, "I want it short and curly," but rather, specify whether you want tight curls, or loose waves, and tell him exactly what you mean by "short." And by all means bring any sketches you may have made (he's not going to judge you as if you were Michelangelo) or pictures you may have clipped from magazines. Ask the stylist—tactfully, please!—if he thinks he can create the style you've just shown him or described to him—not all stylists have the talent or

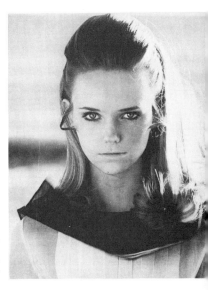

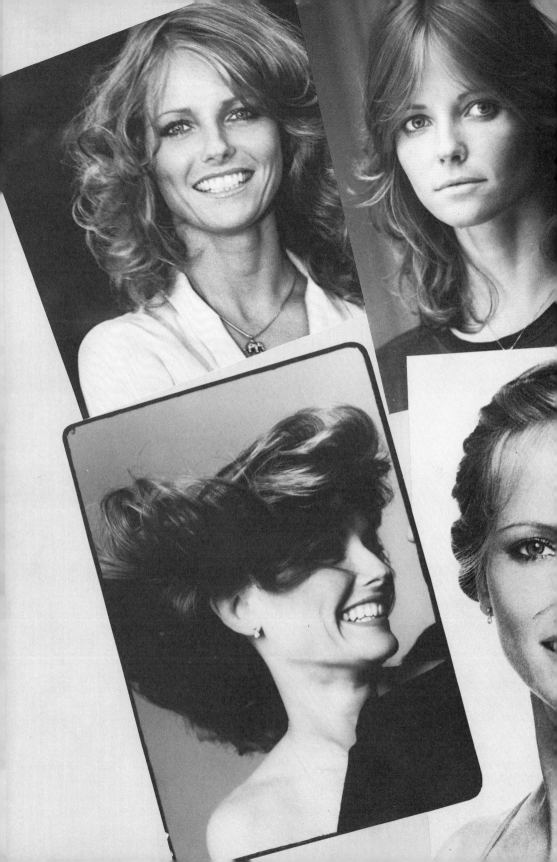

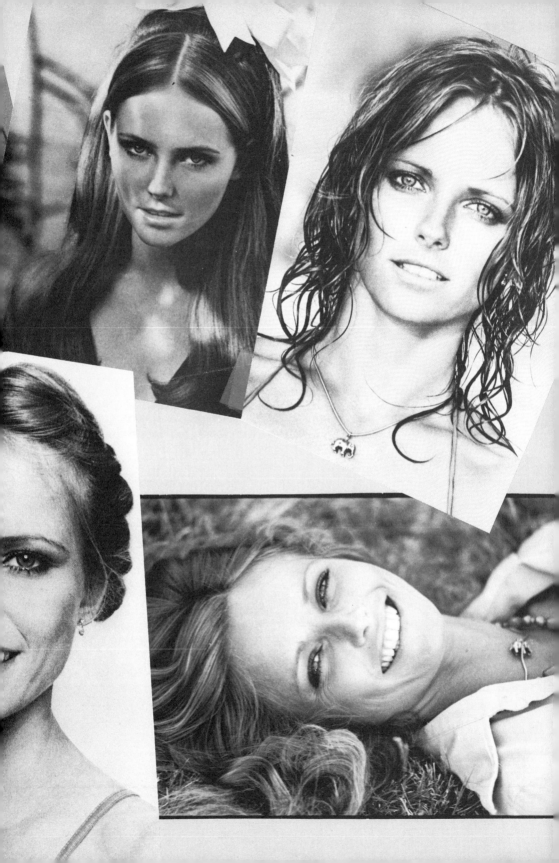

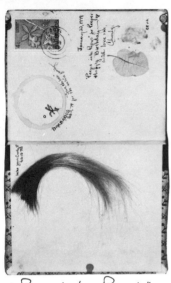

" Peeps into Pepys "

**150**

the training to style for magazine layouts where the models' hair looks eternally perfect instead of just about to disintegrate. Ask him also to check the condition of your hair: Is it fragile, damaged, dry? Can it withstand chemical processing, setting, blow-drying? Before he begins to cut, perm, or color, find out *exactly* what he has in mind. Check out how much care and additional servicing, such as trims and color touch-ups, your new hairstyle will demand. Whenever you don't understand what your stylist is talking about, press him for further details. Your new hairstyle should be the result of a collaboration between you and your stylist and not come as a complete surprise. After many a blunder dies the swan.

When the stylist has finished with you, get him to suggest ways to dress up your new hair for the evening, and ways for you to vary it without changing the basic look. Ask him to show you how to work with your hair at home. If the style requires rollers, curling irons, or blow-drying, you'll need very explicit instructions. Try it yourself with him right there.

During your visit to the salon, pay careful attention to what your stylist is doing with your hair. Too often, women concentrate on telling the stylist the story of their lives, or their friends' lives (gush, simper, rasp!!!), or on reading the latest magazines, and as a result they sometimes emerge with a style they hadn't quite imagined. On rare occasions, it's the stylist who gets carried away on the chitchat. Once, I was having my hair done by a ritzy Paris hairdresser who was so busy gossiping madly to one and all as he curled my hair, that when he took out the sizzling curling iron, a large chunk of my hair came out with it. It was actually smoking—skewered to the iron like a piece of shish-kebab. He continued babbling away, reigning in his own salon, and soon he was turning the damage he'd done me into a spectacularly unfunny story. Needless to say, I was not amused.

(I have a wonderfully bizarre artist friend who never ceases to ask me for locks of my hair to paste into his diary or art collages, and occasionally I oblige him and snip off a piece or two—neither smoking nor skewered, thank you—to the horror of the stylists I work with.)

All of us have gone to a hair salon only to emerge thoroughly depressed. A few years ago, on a whim, I sacrificed my long hair to a cute short layer-cut. The result was disappointingly straight and flat, not at all

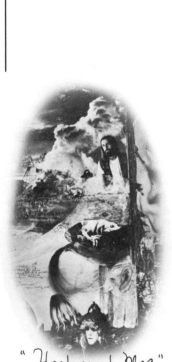

" Fleetwood Mac "

the fluffy picture I'd clipped from a magazine. A mistake, but not a fatal one, for in a few weeks the layers began to grow out again, and the now not so irregular lengths just began to look quite interesting—or so I kept telling myself.

Few new hairstyles are total disasters. You may be disappointed with a hairstyle only because you haven't yet grown accustomed to your new image, or because the new style doesn't instantly and magically and completely transform you. Also, hair goes into "shock" right after it's been cut, and it may be as long as a week before it accepts its new direction. Or maybe your new style looked terrific when you left the salon and then rapidly drooped at home. It takes time to learn to work with a new style successfully. One spongy, curly permanent I was given made me feel like the Bride of Frankenstein. I desperately tried to get my hair to go back to its sleek, smooth look, but it was obstinate and try as I may—and did—I simply could not bend it to my will. I finally decided to accept the fact that I had a bad permanent, and set out to get it to work *for* me. I had a bit snipped off the ends, which tamed the wild curls, and soon my permanent looked okay.

But, if, when all is said and done, you have to admit that your new style really is a disaster, don't let a single bad experience keep you from changing your hairstyle ever again—that could be the most stunting thing, the biggest mistake of all.

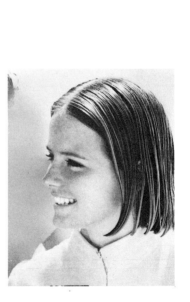

**151**

## WHEN TO CHANGE STYLISTS

If you find a stylist you like, stay with him for a while. It takes even a professional time to get accustomed to your hair type and learn how to work with it—and with you. On the other hand, every stylist has his limitations. If he's been giving you the same old look time after time, year in and year out, you should consider switching to someone more imaginative.

## EXACTLY WHAT IS A GOOD HAIRCUT?

The most important thing in any good hairstyle is the cut.

If your hair is very fine and straight, the best cut for you may be a blunt cut, one the same length all over. This will give your hair body and manageability. The same cut also works well with thick, straight hair.

If your hair is curly or wavy, a slightly layered cut will emphasize the curl without removing too much of it. *Very* curly or frizzy hair should be cut in short layers around the sides and in longer layers in back.

A good stylist will approach the whole problem of your haircut systematically. First he'll divide your hair into sections, and then he'll blunt cut it with scissors. Beware of the stylist who cuts away haphazardly!

Most stylists will wet or dampen your hair before they cut it. When it dries, however, it shrinks and will therefore look shorter than it did when it was wet; your stylist must take this into account when determining your ideal hair length.

A good cut should fall neatly into place after your hair has been washed. You should be able to part it on either side or in the middle and have it fall cleanly. So don't tie yourself down to the same look day after day.

If your hair is layered, it should look even all over, whether it's dry or wet—you shouldn't be able to "see" distinct layers.

## ALTERING THE LOOK OF YOUR BASIC LOOK

Once you have a good basic cut and style, there are many ways to change the mood. There are going to be times when the basic style is just not right for an occasion. I've seen photos of myself in evening clothes with my hair still in its casual daytime look and cringed to realize that it did not mesh with the rest of me. Since nothing can transform your entire appearance faster and more fully than your hair, you'll want to experiment with ways to change its look.

## WHAT YOU SHOULD KNOW ABOUT PERMANENTS

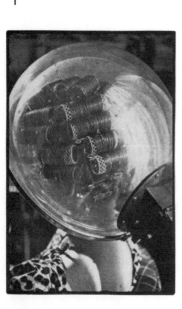

For years I was paranoid about permanents, thanks to the home perms I was given as a child. These once-a-year epics always ended badly. Little me would emerge out of the lotions and curlers with a head of short, crimped frizz. I certainly didn't cut much of a figure in junior high. For weeks after each perm, I would try in vain to grease the fuzz away and to make my shortened hair look longer by combing it down and clipping it to my ears with bobby pins. It must have been then that I decided that as soon as I could afford it I would turn myself over to an expert.

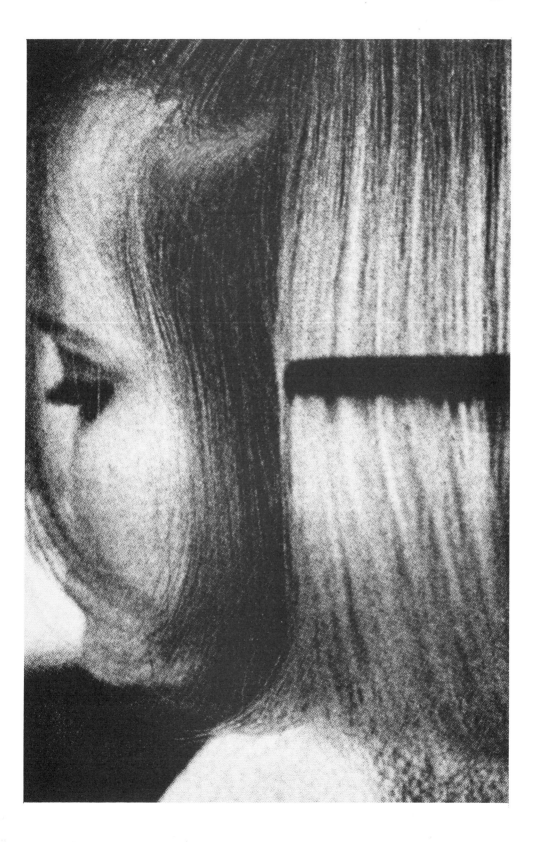

The modern permanent waving process, which is extremely sophisticated, can improve the appearance of many different kinds of hair. A modern perm (also called a "body wave" because of the gentle, relaxed curl it creates) leaves your hair so soft you can step out of the shower and simply shake it dry. The new perms don't leave the sharp indentations between each curl which the old-fashioned perms did; they allow the hair to fall in a natural wave, giving you a style that seems to effortlessly frame your face. Soft, finely textured hair acquires more body with a permanent and holds a set better, while thick, heavy hair acquires a positively beautiful bend. A perm can work a minor miracle on even too-curly hair by removing the topmost frizziness and transforming it into all soft curls.

After a permanent, my hair has shape *and* movement—the same hair that, left to just hang in there, tends to be flat on top and to go limp when I let it grow. A gentle permanent will not produce frizz or fuzz. Sometimes I even forget I have a permanent until I wash or set my hair and realize with grateful amazement how much body and bounce it has.

### WHY BOTHER TO GET
### A PROFESSIONAL PERMANENT?

The permanent wave process is complicated to a degree. If any one of the number of steps it entails is carried out irresponsibly, your permanent will end up frizzy, loose, and limp—a far cry from the shape you'd been counting on it to assume. Perms today are done with a new acid-based type of wave lotion, which breaks the chemical bonds that determine the shape of each hair. These new lotions can't destroy your hair, but it takes an expert to know just what kind of lotion will work best with your hair type and, even more important, how long it should stay on. After the lotion is applied, the hair is set in a curl or wave pattern. Again, it takes a professional to correctly space the curlers and to determine what size they should be to create a particular style. Finally, the hair is neutralized with yet another chemical, which makes it possible for the restructured hair to remain in the shape of a curl. If you can afford it, have your permanent done in a really good salon. However, if you do go ahead and try to give yourself a home permanent, proceed with caution: Read and follow the directions very, very carefully. And if your home perm fails, don't try it again.

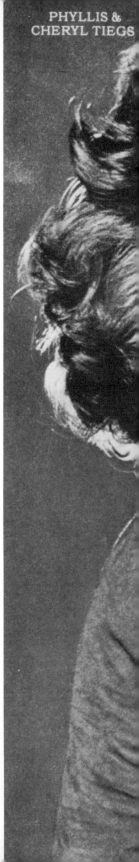

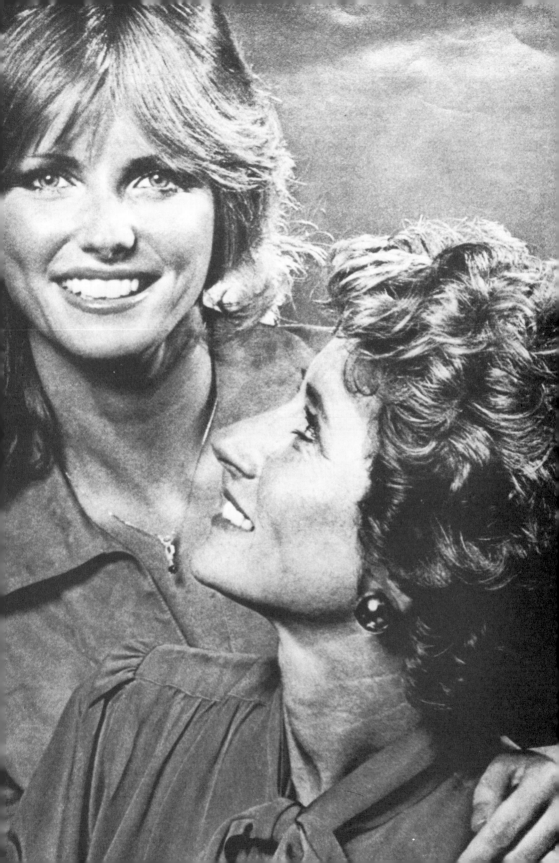

## THE AFTER-CARE OF A PERM

A permanent should be trimmed regularly if you want it to continue to look good. A bit of dryness is bound to creep into the last eighth inch of hair that's been permed, but if you just remove those ends the entire perm will get a big lift. If your hair seems too frizzy after a perm, a trim also will tame it down. With frequent trims you can get away with having to have a permanent only every six months or so.

## STRAIGHTENING YOUR HAIR: SHOULD YOU DO IT?

Wouldn't you know it: women lucky enough to have naturally curly hair often want to have it straightened. Just why, I always wonder, when curly hair can be brought under control by means of a good cut, and extremely curly hair can be greatly enhanced by a short layered style. If, however, you do decide to have your hair chemically straightened, take your head to a good salon. The chemicals used in reversing a curl are very powerful and should under no circumstances be handled by an amateur. A bad straightening job can cause your hair to break off at the scalp. Try taming any unruly curls by pushing the damp hair into waves, securing them with clips, and letting your hair dry—to use my favorite adverb—*naturally*.

## COLORING YOUR HAIR IN: RED, WHITE, BLUE?

A new hair color can pick up glints and flecks in your eyes and tones in your skin, dramatize your hair with deep, rich shades, or cool it down to a subtly sophisticated hue. Streaking can approximate the lightening powers of the summer sun to frame your face with lighter shades. Hair color can also act as a conditioner, thickening each strand for greater body and manageability. Color rinses lightly coat the shaft of your hair till you shampoo them right out, and semi-permanent tints permeate the hair shaft for as long as a month. Both of these techniques are good for temporarily deepening the shade of your hair or adding attractive highlights. If you are intent on actually changing your hair color, a permanent tint that really penetrates the hair shaft is necessary.

Definitely leave any major and drastic color change to a professional colorist. He will have the know-how to select and blend the right tones of the tint with your own hair color, so the hair shade you wind up with is a subtle combination of *natural* tones that is also going to look good with your skin.

Hair coloring can certainly be a success at home. The colors shown on the packages are indications of what the colors would look like on white hair. The packages have a panel showing or telling what the color will look like on different shades of hair. Read and follow the instructions carefully and you can achieve the look you want with the greatest of ease.

Take the time to analyze your skin tone before you change your hair color. If your complexion is very pale, avoid black or any harsh color. Olive-skinned, dark-eyed women make unconvincing blondes. And women with glowing, ruddy complexions are making a big mistake when they opt for a red or auburn hair color. If you are going gray—extreme hair colors will invariably make you look older than you are. A good rule of thumb is: Select a subtle tone, a shade lighter than your natural color, or one as close to it as possible. If you're a brunette who believes that blondes have more fun, have fun trying it.

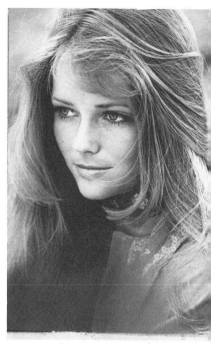

Streaking can be natural

If it's a radical color change you're mulling over (from brunette to blond, or black to red, for example), calculate the time and money it's going to take to maintain the new shade. If you can't afford salon touch-ups, either reconsider your decision or get your colorist to give you instructions for retouching your hair yourself.

The front of your hair just near the hairline is usually a bit lighter than the rest. If you want to lighten your hair a shade, try matching the new color to this part of your hair.

Always deep-condition your hair for several weeks before and after a permanent color change.

And this above all: Wait at least four weeks between coloring sessions; and be careful when you use one color dye on top of another that it doesn't produce an unexpected color change.

## HENNA

Made from a plant that grows in the Middle East, henna is one of the oldest of hair dyes. The princesses of Egypt and Persia used this organic, nontoxic hair

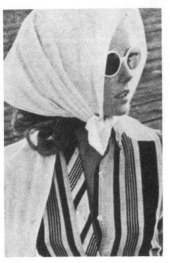

coloring agent to condition and color their hair, and if it was good enough for *them*. . . . Henna, when used properly, adds a real sheen. It also coats each strand, and gives your hair strength and body. Natural henna adds no color but brings out natural highlights. But, as with most anything, improper use can be damaging. Blondes and those with light-tinted hair should be particularly careful.

## HAIR CARE: WHO CARES?

No style will look attractive on you if your hair is bedraggled looking. But if it's well-nourished and looks well-groomed, almost any carefully thought-out style will look flattering.

## SHAMPOOING

When I was a little girl I washed my hair once a week only, because my mother put great stock in the old myth that frequent shampooing damages hair by depriving it of needed oils. There are in fact no rules that dictate how often you should shampoo, except the basic one of common sense: If your hair is dirty, wash it. Only oily hair, or hair that tends to become limp and separate a day or so after washing, should be shampooed very often—in some cases, every day. Dry or dull hair requires less shampooing. If you live in a city rather than a suburb or the country, it may be a good idea to shampoo fairly often, given the pollutants in the environment.

## WHICH SHAMPOO IS THE ONE FOR YOU?

Try not to cringe, but the best shampoo is a mild, *detergent* shampoo formulated especially for your hair type. "Detergent" is a harsh word, I know, conjuring up as it does sinkfuls of soaking dishes, but it's the best ingredient for cutting through the grease and grime in your hair. Most shampoos contain it. Like many of the other ingredients in shampoo, it passes over your hair shaft ever so briefly, en route to being washed down the drain. Acid, or pH-balanced shampoos, lock moisture into the hair, and are good for normal as well as dry hair. However, they may not be powerful enough to clean oily hair, and might leave it looking dull. Nor will protein, egg, and balsam shampoos do the job for oily hair that they will for fine, thin, or limp

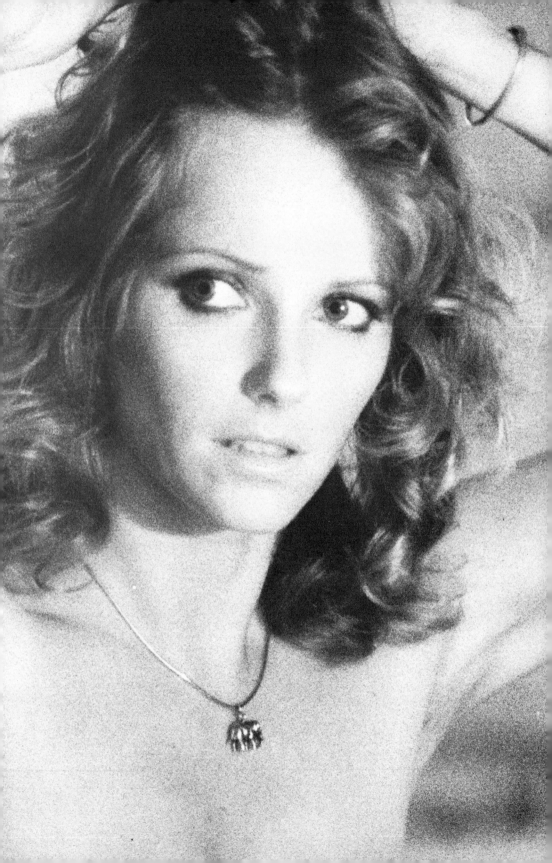

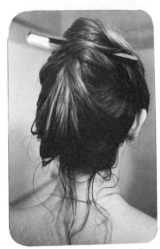

*No shower cap?*
*— Use a toothbrush*

hair. So if your hair is oily, try to choose a shampoo containing *lemon*.

I certainly shopped around a lot before I hit on the shampoo I now use. It's a trial-and-error kind of thing.

## HOW TO SHAMPOO: GENTLY, GENTLY DOWN THE DRAIN

Always handle your hair gently. Massaging the soap into your scalp with your fingertips will stimulate the roots of your hair and scalp. And be sure to rinse out every little trace of shampoo, which if you're not careful can leave a dull, drying film on your hair. Don't lather on great gobs of shampoo, because the more of it you use the harder it will be to rinse it all away. At one time in my adult life, I was using shampoo by the handful! Not surprisingly—except, come to think of it, it *was* a big surprise to me—my hair began to dry out. So I decided to be a good girl and obey the instructions on the label for a change, to wit: "Massage one half-teaspoon of shampoo into your hair." I learned the thorny way that a lot is not always better than a little. Also, hot water doesn't necessarily rinse the soap out of your hair effectively. Follow it with a cool rinse that also stimulates scalp circulation. If you shampoo your hair every day, lather once only. But if your hair is really dirty, you may need to give it two separate lathers. Never brush or yank at your hair with a comb when it's wet. And disentangle knots with your fingers before you comb—but gently, gently.

## GOOD CONDITIONING

Conditioners help protect your hair from all the factors that never cease conspiring against it—sun, wind, pollution, chlorine, central heating, not to mention blow-dryers, hot curlers, and the alkaline chemicals used in permanent wave and color processing.

No conditioner can actually repair damaged hair, as some of the advertisements would have you believe. Once an end is split or a hair shaft becomes porous and brittle, the only way to cure it is to cut it off and let a new hair replace it.

Conditioners temporarily coat the hair shaft, making it appear thicker. They also fill in the rough surface of the hair cuticle, so the hair seems softer and smoother. The cream conditioners used after shampooing untangle hair, make it easier to comb, and

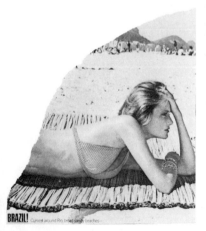

BRAZIL! Curved around Rio, broad sandy beaches

tame dry, flyaway tresses. But if your hair is oily or damaged, keep clear of cream conditioners; with their alkaline nature, they can make oily hair limp. If you have very oily hair, a home remedy might just do the trick—add a quarter cup of lemon juice or cider vinegar to a quart of water as a final rinse. I use a special conditioner that brings out my blond highlights, which I apply after I wash my hair and let it sink in. If you fail to rinse conditioners out thoroughly, they'll leave a dull film.

## DEEP-CONDITIONING TREATMENTS

Dry, damaged, or chemically processed hair should be deep-conditioned often. Protein conditioners, which you should leave on your hair for twenty minutes and/ or use with heat, and hot oil treatments penetrate and coat the hair shaft, making it softer and much more pliable. You can make a protein conditioner at home by mixing two egg yolks with one tablespoon of sesame oil (not exactly my idea of a box lunch); work it into your hair, and then cover it with a hot, damp towel. For a homemade oil treatment, heat some plain olive or safflower oil; divide your clean, dry hair into sections; comb the oil through; wrap your hair in a plastic bag; and sit under a bonnet dryer for between twenty and thirty minutes. To get the oil out, apply an undiluted shampoo to your dry hair, lather, then rinse thoroughly.

Oily hair does not benefit from deep-conditioning treatments. But if it's only your scalp that's oily, and the ends of your hair seem dry, deep-condition the ends only. (It makes sense, right?)

## BRUSHING

Should you brush your hair the fabled one hundred strokes a day? Yes—if you enjoy a good exercise in futility, and like to live dangerously to boot. Too much brushing can aggravate your hair and scalp and cause your hair to thin right out. If your hair is dry or already damaged in any way, go very lightly with the hairbrush.

If your hair is in generally good condition, however, an occasional brushing will stimulate blood circulation in the scalp, do away with superficial dandruff, and get the natural hair oils moving from the base of the scalp to the ends of the hair shaft, where they're often

161

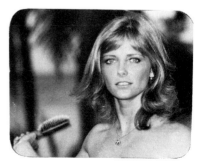

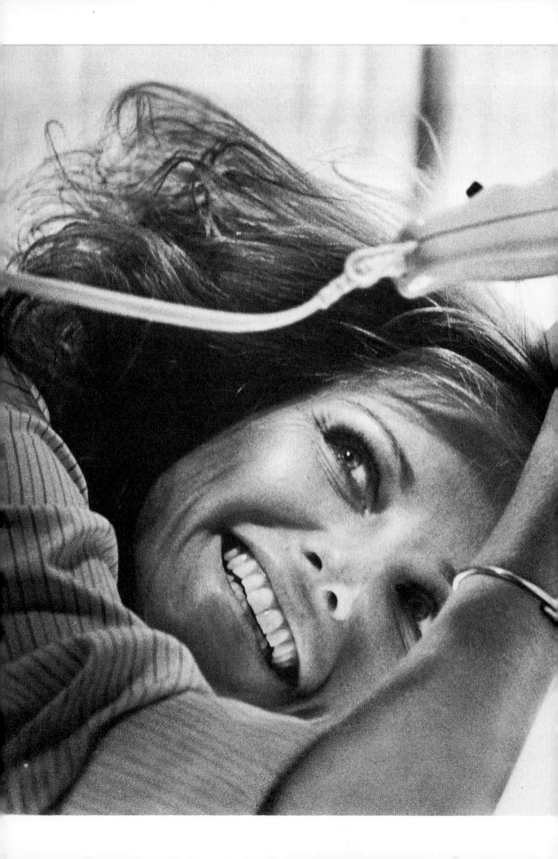

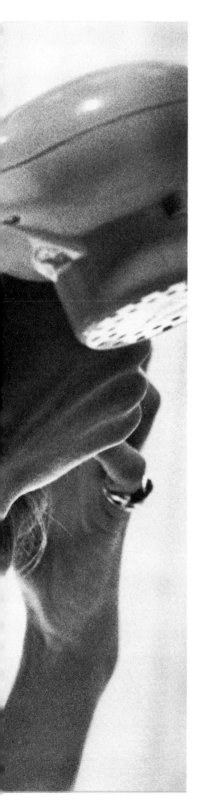

needed more desperately. Since brushing loosens dirt, making it easier to remove, a good time to brush is just before you wash your hair. I brush the underside of my hair by bending over and throwing my hair forward, so it'll look full and flowing. You'll want a good hairbrush, preferably one combining natural boar and soft plastic bristles on a cushioning foam base. Never use a brush with nylon bristles—they tear at the hair and damage it.

## DRYERS! HOT ROLLERS! CURLING IRONS!!!

There aren't two opinions: electrical appliances do give hair a glamorous lift but (and it's a pretty big "but"), if you use them too often you may be risking your hair's health. I try to let my hair dry naturally as often as possible. In fact, the only time I resort to hot rollers and curling irons is before special occasions.

Say your hair does look best blow-dried, then go ahead, but set your dryer on "cool" (it's the heat— along with the blast of air—that dries your hair out). The more modern dryers have an adjustable power dial that allows you to control the wattages you send to your hair. For serious drying, a 1,000-watt setting works best, but for styling and touch-ups, 750 or even 500 watts will do. To blow-dry safely and effectively, hold the dryer about six inches away from your head, moving it as you brush continuously, and taking care not to overheat any one section of your hair or scalp.

Hot rollers are wonderful time-savers, yes, but they too can damage your hair if you use them too often. The type that works with steam adds more moisture to hair than the dry-heat types does, but may not be as effective in humid weather, when your hair already contains plenty of moisture. Leave hot rollers in for only three minutes, then let the curls cool before combing them out.

Most modern curling irons are Teflon-coated and have a thermostat so they can't overheat and sear your hair. They should be used only on dry hair; if they're used on wet hair, they may make the curls too tight. Curling irons, like all other forms of heating equipment, must be used in moderation.

## HELPING YOUR HAIR FROM THE INSIDE OUT

Truly healthy hair begins beneath the scalp, with the roots you don't see. These roots are nourished through the circulatory system, and just like the rest of your body, they benefit from a good diet and plenty of exercise. The hair shaft is basically composed of a protein substance, so a diet rich (but not too rich) in protein will help form strong, shiny hair. It can be said that good hair, like good skin, is the end result of a balanced diet, one full of vitamins and minerals.

I've made this list of time-saving tips for styling and caring for hair:

## SPRAY AND PUFF

To perk up curly hair or a permanent that looks as if it had just been run over, lightly mist your hair with the same spray bottle you use to mist your houseplants. Your curls will spring instantly, abundantly back into shape. Use your fingers to fluff them out.

## SUN AND OIL TREATMENT

Not that many people know this but overexposure to the sun can do as much damage to your hair as to your skin. However, if you know how, you can utilize the sun's rays to give your hair what amounts to a deep-conditioning oil treatment. Before you go to the beach, simply comb a conditioner or some sweet almond or coconut oil into your hair. The oil will protect your hair from the sun's drying rays, while the sun helps the oil penetrate your hair shaft. This is the method that women in India and countries with a similar climate have always used to keep their dark hair sleek and shining.

## HOMEMADE BALSAM RINSES

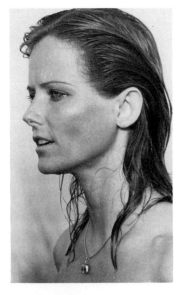

An old-fashioned way to bring out the highlights in your hair is to rinse it with a homemade herbal brew. The recipe is anything but elaborate: just steep a quarter cup of rosemary (if your hair is dark; if it's light, substitute camomile flowers) in a quart of boiling water and let it sit till the mixture has a strong color and aroma. Then cool and strain it. Use the aromatic result as the final rinse for your hair. A brew of dried nettles also adds luster and body to hair—improbable as that sounds.

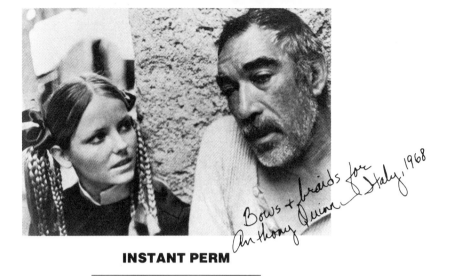

*Bows + braids for Italy, 1968*
*Anthony Quinn*

## INSTANT PERM

If you'd like to try a curly look without subjecting your-self to processing chemicals, braid your damp hair in about eight braids all over your head just before going to bed. In the morning, undo the braids and marvel at your fluffy, wavy instant perm!

## BRUSHING AND SPRAYING

Personally, I hate the look of stiff, sprayed hair that doesn't budge an inch. I've found a good use for hair-spray, however, After I remove the hot curlers and brush hair into place, I spray my hair, *then* brush out most of the spray half an hour later. What the spray does is accustom my hair to the shape I want and also adds body, and brushing it out does away with that depressing unnatural look.

## RELAXING CURLS

Whenever I set my hair in rollers, I make sure I re-move them *before* I get dressed for a night out. That way, I give my curls a chance to relax, and I also get a chance to see the way my hair is actually going to look for the rest of the night: I mean, like can I live with it for five hours?

## MISTAKES PEOPLE MAKE

### Wearing a Too-Extravagant Hairstyle

Some women persist in making the near-fatal error of sporting a mass of frizzy curls or—every bit as bad—an over-elaborate hairdo, which I jokingly call the

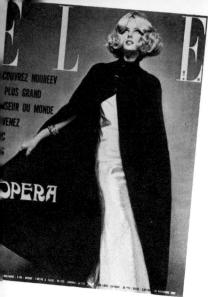

"important" hairdo, that overpowers rather than frames their face. Others crop their hair too short, over-henna it, or streak it a most peculiar shade. Xandra Rhodes can get away with wearing green or purple hair, and so can David Bowie, but we're not all famous fashion designers and punk rockers. Don't adopt a deliberately offbeat style to make an outrageous statement that doesn't become you. You want people to notice your hair because it's an integral part of your total attractive look—not because it's overstyled, overpowering, over zany, or just plain weird.

### Changing Hairstyles for the Wrong Reason

It's a mistake to change your hairstyle because you are feeling insecure or depressed. There's a good chance that if you change your hair hoping to improve your state of mind you'll just saddle yourself with another disaster.

I used to go to a lot of trouble to reproduce whatever "latest" hairstyle had caught my fancy or fired my imagination—completely oblivious to how it would look on me. Well, you live and *maybe* you learn. But I do know what I'm talking about when I say: the latest hairstyle should always be the style that looks best on you.

### Grooming Your Hair for All the World to See

Nothing can ruin—or, at the very least, tarnish—your image faster than combing or grooming your hair in public. Because I'm always in a rush—with me, it's always one giant step forward and two baby steps backward—I often have to leave the house with my hair still damp from the shower, but I always make sure that the final combing takes place in the privacy of a ladies' room or, failing that, the semi-privacy of a cab. And there's absolutely no excuse to ever be seen in curlers outside your own house—they make everyone look sort of wired-for-sound, and somewhat freakish.

### Sleeping on Curlers

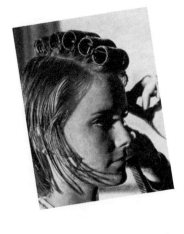

Every night during my teens I would set my hair, put out the lights, and lay down to sleep on the bumpy curlers. Had I only seen that great movie *All About Eve*, I could have said the famous Bette Davis line to myself instead of my boring prayers, "Fasten your seatbelts, it's going to be a *bumpy* ride." I shudder to think how fragile and brittle that bad practice must have made my hair. It's amazing how few clangorous nightmares I had.

### Butchering Your Own Hair

If you're one of those who must "do it yourself," restrict your cutting efforts to snipping an eighth of an inch from the ends between salon visits. Just about the most frustrating thing to a stylist is having to deal with the ragged ends and holes caused by a bad haircut. Haircutting is not as easy as it looks. It takes a good stylist *years* to learn his trade. And don't entrust your scissors to a well-meaning friend, either.

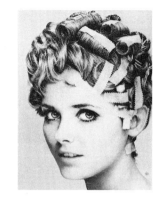

### Crash Dieting

Here's a sure way to damage your hair (as well as the rest of your body): Deprive yourself of the nutrients you need by going on a good crash diet. Each hair on your head has a natural growing and resting phase; it's during the resting phase that it falls out, soon to be replaced by a new hair. If your diet's too poor to provide your hair with the fertilizer it needs in order to grow (about 800 calories per day) your hair will be "hungry," and as many as half the hairs on your head may go into their resting phase at the same time (as opposed to the usual ten percent), with the result that your hair fallout rate will increase dramatically—and visibly!

### Styling Hair in Tight Braids, Chignons, Ponytails

Any style that places a disproportionate amount of pressure on one part of your hair will eventually cause it to thin out. So save ponytails, corn-rows, tight chignons for your temporary look. Variety is the answer here as elsewhere.

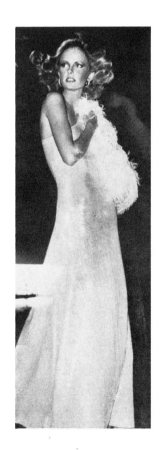

### Fighting Your Hair All the Way

I have a cowlick that I can't lick. It's been the grief of quite a few stylists (and given others an actual sick headache). Over the years my friendly cowlick has eluded all manner of clipping, combing, and nudging. Believe me, the only way to go is *with it*—accept the texture and direction of your hair. By all means, strive to improve the look of it by means of curlers, tints, perms, and new cuts, but don't fight your natural, God-given hair to the death.

Because, take it from me, it's a losing battle.

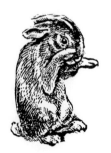

# 6

## Making Up to Yourself: Facing Up to Your Face

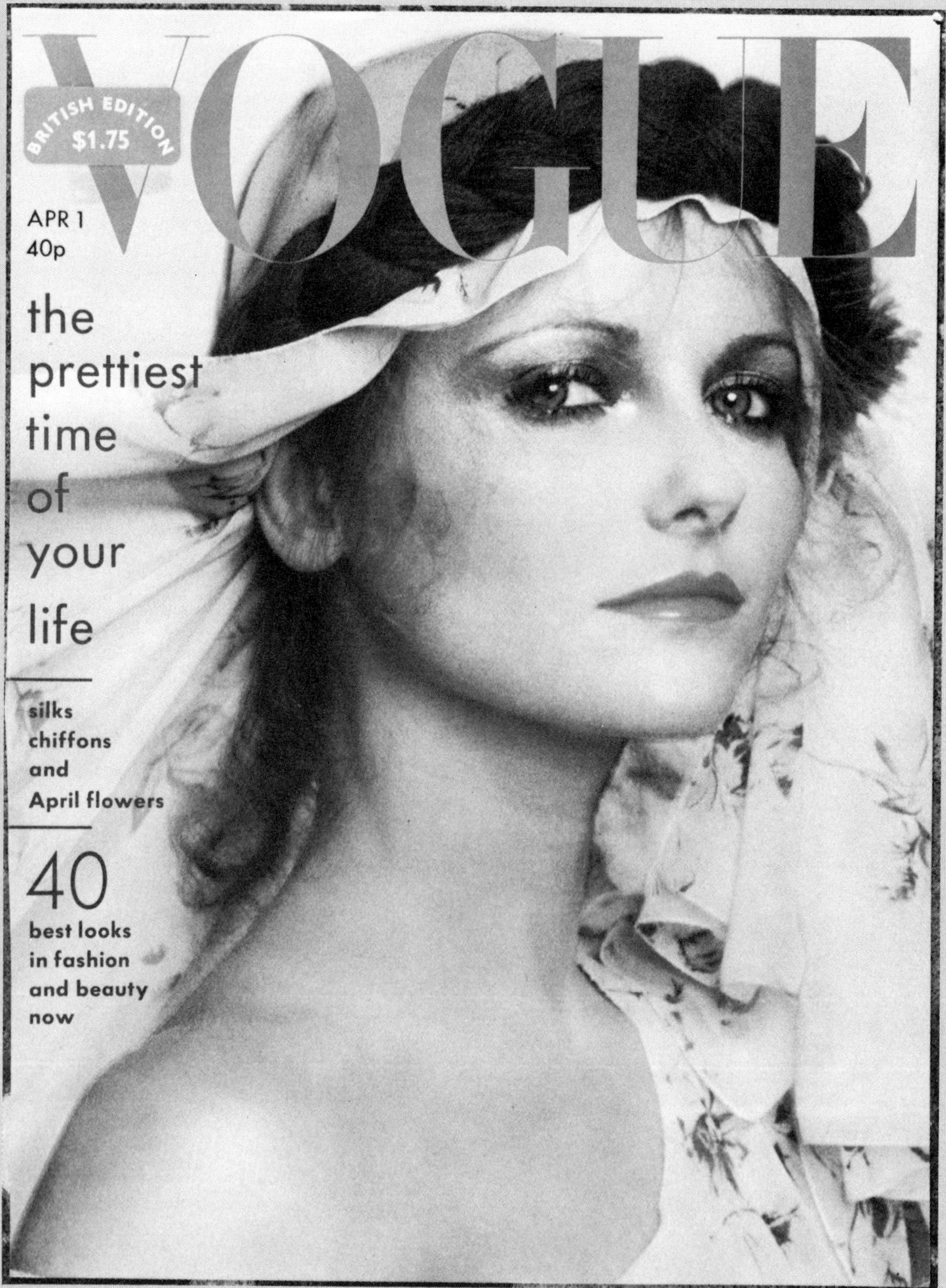

# VOGUE

APR 1
40p

the
prettiest
time
of
your
life

silks
chiffons
and
April flowers

40
best looks
in fashion
and beauty
now

eauty is never certain, it's highly conditional. Our assets are only lent to us. We *have* to pay attention to them. If only because they are always being assessed—by others as well as ourselves! In Japan recently I picked up a novel called *Snow Country* by Yasunari Kawabata, a Nobel-Prize winner. The heroine, Komako, is a country geisha in a Japanese hot-springs resort. I was impressed by how the author's style communicates "the joy of the knowing eye, of the sensitive skin, of the ear, the nose and the tongue." I certainly learned something about the whole procedure of beauty from Kawabata's description of his heroine:

*The high, thin nose was a little lonely, a little sad, but the bud of her lips opened and closed smoothly, like a beautiful circle of leeches. When she was silent her lips seemed always to be moving. Had they wrinkles or cracks, or had their color been less fresh, they would have struck one as unwholesome, but they were never anything but smooth and shining. The line of her eyelids neither rose nor fell. As if for some special reason, it drew its way straight across her face. There was something faintly comical about the effect, but the short, thick hair of her eyebrows sloped gently down to enfold the line discreetly. There was nothing remarkable about the outline of her round, slightly aquiline face. With her skin like white porcelain coated over a faint pink, and her throat still girlish, not yet filled out, the impression she gave was above all one of cleanness, not quite one of real beauty.*

Here is a woman who has seen to it that her face mirrors her considerable understanding of the world. Looking into the mirror, she would not be like a character in another novel who said that she felt a stranger to her own face.

At the other extreme, I've just finished Dirk Bogarde's fascinating memoir, *Snakes & Ladders*. He's always been one of my favorite actors, ever since I saw him in *The Servant* in a pokey little art-movie house outside of Alhambra. When Dirk describes the filming of the death scene in Thomas Mann's classic, *Death in Venice*, under the great Italian director Visconti, I couldn't help thinking how the poor pain of all those made-up hours would serve as a cautionary tale, at

*The inspiration behind the VOGUE cover was — coincidentally — one of my very favorite books — "The Wilder Shores of Love". I imagined myself as Isabelle Burton — entering Mecca — exploring Africa in the 1800's.*

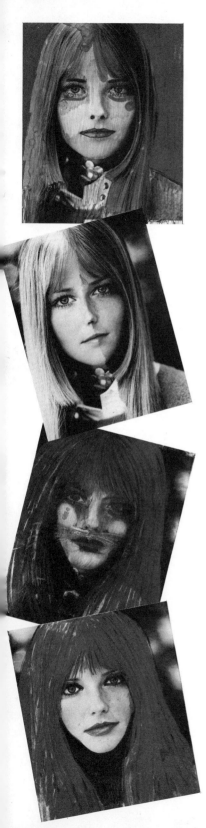

least as far as this chapter's concerned—and possibly beyond.

*I noticed, casually, one day, that some of the troupe . . . were walking about wearing neat little squares of white paint, no bigger than a postage stamp. I didn't pay very much attention, but after three or four days, and an ever-increasing amount of little white squares . . . I asked. . . . They were testing some kind of make-up.*

*. . . of all the things which I had to face in the film the thing which frightened me most was the actual, final, death scene . . . Clearly the moment was upon us. They were testing special make-up because the one I would have to use must be a total death mask: it was to crack apart slowly, symbolizing decay, age, ruin . . . But I kept silent, as was my habit, and merely watched with mounting terror the daily proliferation of little white patches among the troupe. Whatever they were using . . . was going to be both unpleasant, and possibly from the amount of care being taken, dangerous.*

*. . . In the make-up room Visconti was quiet, firm, and very gentle. ". . . you are sick now, and old; re-member what Mann has said, you will have lips as ripe as strawberries . . . the dye from your hair will run . . . your poor face will crack, and then you will die . . . I tell you all this because when you have the make-up on your face you will not be able to speak, it will be dead as a mask . . . we only do one take for that reason . . . it is hard like a plaster."*

Translated into real life, the moral of Dirk's macabre experience may be that the last thing you want to present to the world is the death mask of makeup.

If you want your appearance to serve you, so that when you look in the mirror it's not an enemy you're facing, you will have to learn the craft of making up. If you apply makeup correctly, it can dramatize your face. Cheek color, eye color, and lip color can all work together to emphasize your best features—adding just the right, sometimes barely perceptible, touch of freshness and get-it-togetherness.

But if you don't take the time to learn how to refurbish yourself, then it's going to be, in Virginia Tiger's clever phrase from her useful book, *Everywoman*, "combat in the cosmetic zone"—and war is war, and "beauty can kill. Yet it is a university as well as a jungle."

We don't have to accept our sallow skin and dank hair. With know-how we can subdue them till we're at the very least, presentable.

So why do many women persist in turning their faces into disaster areas? Too much makeup, coarsely, clumsily, or too thickly plastered on, may make you look garish or artificial. Too little makeup, or none at all, may leave you looking lusterless, definitely on the dull side, just about to be eclipsed by everything and everyone.

Believe me, you don't want to play at making-up. It's a very serious business, and the stakes are high.

If you want your face to come to your aid as you go about your day, the first thing you should do is ask yourself a few hard questions—and not be afraid to answer them. Well, you want to hold up your head and glitter, don't you?

■ *Do you look at your daytime makeup in natural light before you leave the house in the morning?*

■ *Do you apply lipstick with a brush?*

■ *Do you make an effort to use an eyeshadow that matches the color of the clothes you have on?*

■ *Before you buy makeup base, do you test the color on your hand?*

■ *Do you conceal dark shadows under your eyes with a light-colored concealing cream?*

■ *Do you "finish" your evening makeup by applying translucent powder with a brush over your foundation to prevent shine?*

■ *Are you one who believes that makeup base clogs your pores and should be worn only on special occasions?*

■ *How do you keep your eye makeup from slipping? By applying a neutral foundation to your eyelids, or what?*

■ *Do you blend your eyeliner with the tip of your finger?*

■ *Has anyone ever complimented you on your makeup? Were they empty compliments?*

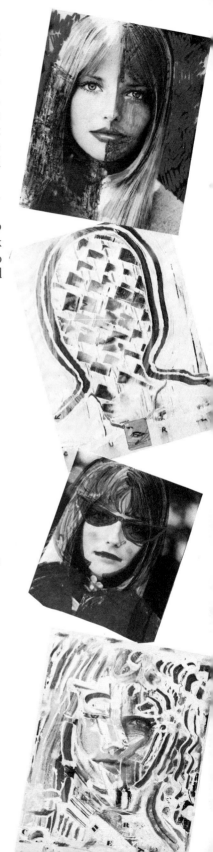

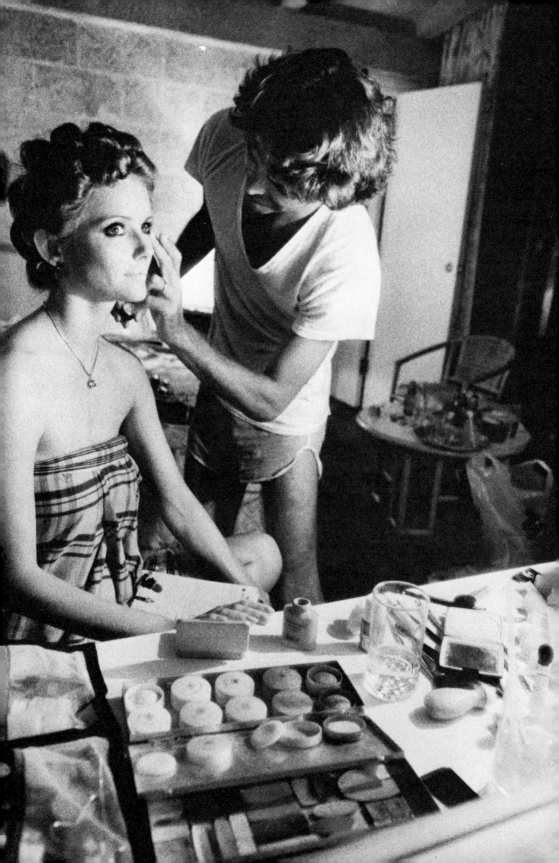

Just show me the face that doesn't need decorating, or doctoring. For models, it's a life and death affair. It's makeup that sets the mood of the clothes we wear, creates a kind of weather for them. It's makeup that heightens the illusion in all those fashion photographs you see. I call it "the art that conceals art" because when it's been done well, you hardly notice it.

In my career I've been very lucky to know and work with some great makeup artists like Way Bandy and François Ilnseher. I've studied the types of makeup they use on my face and the come-and-go of all kinds of powders, shadows, and pastes—and I've studied how they put them on. A lot of this knowledge I save exclusively for the short life of my appearance before the cameras. The makeup that gives my face a vibrant look in a photograph is much too dramatic for real life. I've had to learn patiently how to modify and tone down the makeup techniques used in the studio.

Perhaps the most serious mistake a woman can make in her appearance is to wear too much makeup. Instead of giving her the freshness of whatever age she is, it tends to make her look older and less—rather than more—sophisticated. It's just another form of dishonesty—if you ask me—and one that boomerangs. And *men* don't like it when the makeup gets too thick. In fact, they often complain that they find a heavy cosmetic look unkissable and untouchable. They have to search for the buried treasure: the real girl stirring beneath the plaster. Too much labor, too much *toil*, can actually be the death not only of a woman's looks but of her love life. I'm not saying men don't want and appreciate the transformation—they do, they just don't want to see it, smell it, meet it in your face. They don't want to even hear about the machinery. When they look at you, they want to see a face, and not that fatal mask of cosmetics.

But don't make the opposite mistake of going totally "natural," and not wearing any makeup at all. There are women today who feel that makeup is just too much trouble to put on, or else that it's too "traditional." (Maybe so. But then, so is the whole idea of looking charming!) They fail to take advantage of all that makeup can do for their faces. Oh there are a few women who can get away with not wearing any makeup whatsoever—the ones with the startling coloring, fire-bright eyes, and flawlessly glowing skin —you know them, all five of them, and there comes a time when even they . . . Almost everyone else,

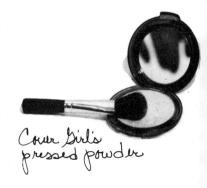

*Cover Girl's pressed powder*

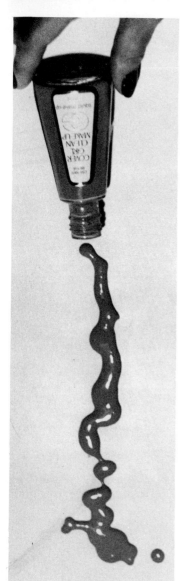

though, can benefit from the addition of color and contrast.

I love a natural look, but it's a rare day when I leave the house without a touch of foundation, blusher, maybe some mascara, and lip gloss. Because I know what even a smidgeon of makeup can do for me: it's the difference between the dog days and the dogwood days. To see a brighter version of my own face in the mirror lifts my spirits and swells my self-confidence when I'm tired or fed up.

## BACK TO THE BASICS OR FORWARD TO??

Most people think that models lug a veritable steamer trunk of cosmetics around with them. Not true! I have a battered old striped tote bag containing the most essential makeup products only—and some of these products I've used for years.

Sure it's fun to change makeup colors every now and again, and it's always fun to experiment with new products. The new cosmetics are lighter and sheerer, but I just don't think it's necessary to buy every cosmetic that comes on the market (it's expensive and time-consuming, too).

Whenever you do buy makeup, do yourself a favor and test it first. Most department stores and pharmacies have samples you can try. Many brands of makeup may look the same but they're made from different recipes; once you've applied them to your skin, they diffuse their mystic attributes. And keep it on while you shop, then look in the mirror—hard (you have to be prepared to be self-critical)—and if you *still* like what it's doing for you, *then* buy it.

Another thing I've learned is that the inexpensive brands can be just as effective as the ones that come in those elaborate containers.

Now back to that old striped tote bag. Here are the makeup items I always carry:

## MAKEUP BASE OR FOUNDATION

Foundation doesn't clog your pores, as many people mistakenly think. Even when I'm outdoors I usually wear a light coat of makeup base: it protects skin from the sun, wind, and city soot. It also evens out skin tone without camouflaging it. A natural skin tone is never a single, consistent shade. Your foundation—*if* you apply it skillfully—should allow some of your natural skin color to show through. Heavy makeup base tends to accumulate in the creases of your face, so don't use foundation to "conceal" wrinkles.

### How to Use It

If you apply moisturizer before foundation, you can spread the base on more evenly. I prefer to let my fingers do the walking—I want to feel where the base is going and work it into all the little out-of-the-way dust-bitten corners. A moist cosmetic sponge is a good tool for applying a super-light coat of base; it wipes some off while some more goes on.

### How to Choose It

If your skin is oily, you should probably use a water based or emulsion-type foundation containing little or no oil. But beware: some water-based foundations are so sheer they may not be giving you the cover you need. Dry-skinned women are much better off using an oil-based foundation. Some makeup bases contain moisturizers, special skin medications, and sun screens as well. Foundations also come in gels, in foams that feel practically weightless, and in cake formulations that are too heavy for that sheer natural look I like so much. You should always try a makeup base before buying it; and don't use your hand to test (the skin color of your hand couldn't be more different from that of your face); instead, apply the sample to the skin of your jaw, where you can see easily how the base blends with the skin on both your face and your neck. Most women prefer a base that's close to their natural skin color. An ivory-colored or neutral base is good for removing redness at the base of the nose and for disguising differences in skin tone. But don't hide your ego behind a foundation. You don't want it to completely change your skin color, you just want it to blend with your own skin.

### Powder Power

I dust my face with powder to set the makeup and give it a good matte finish. If you don't like the idea of dusting your whole face, do just the forehead, chin, and nose, the "T-zone," which has a tendency to get all shiny. I use one of those big soft sable cosmetic brushes that lightly waft the powder over my face.

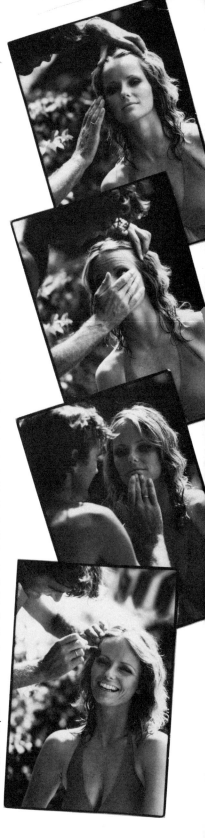

Whether you use a pressed cake or a loose powder, choose the kind that won't interfere with the tone of your other makeup.

## CHEEK-TO-CHEEK COLOR

In almost every interview I've ever done, I've been asked what's the one cosmetic I would take with me if I knew I was going to be stranded on a desert island, the one cosmetic I would rescue from a burning house. And I always answer that the one thing I'd grab for—vanity of vanities!—is my blusher. To me, the most indispensable item in that old striped bag is cheek color—it adds a real glow to the face that to most of us, alas, doesn't come all that naturally.

Makeup experts haven't been exactly shy in recommending techniques for applying blusher. We've all been inundated and confused by the elaborate crescents, arcs, and circles illustrated in the magazines. For me, the simplest and most effective—not to say, most instinctive—way of applying cheek color is to put it on top of the cheekbone, right where the sun would naturally tinge my face. Most of us don't happen to have very prominent cheekbones. Feel for them with your fingers (just light a candle and pray they're going to be there), or suck in your cheeks to make them stand out like Katharine Hepburn's or Faye Dunaway's. Now blend the blush along the line of the cheekbone out toward your temples. If your cream rouge is stiff and hard to handle, apply it with a damp cosmetic sponge, or with slightly moist fingers. Powdered blusher can be applied with the sable cosmetic brush. Liquid cheek color you can apply just to the cheekbone, or to the whole face for a charged but subtle glow.

### How to Choose It

Cheek color comes in cream, rouge, powdered blusher, liquid, gel, and pencil. I prefer a cream-type rouge for day—it adds an extra shine—and powdered blush-on for night. The trouble with powders is they can look obvious and grainy in natural daylight, and shiny creams and gels can look oily under artificial lighting. Powdered blush-on goes better with the powder you use in finishing your evening look. Liquid and gel-type cheek colors are nice for daytime too, because they're light and natural and blend so nicely with your skin.

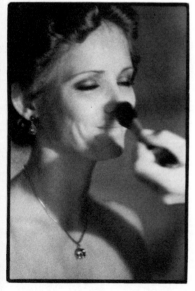

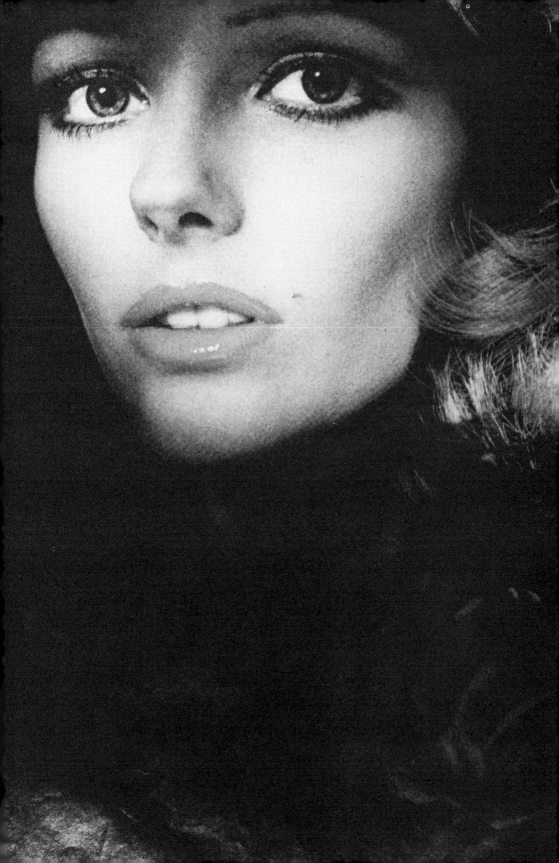

According to that wizard François, who has done my face for so many modeling assignments, I'm beginning to think he knows it better than I do, there are basically two skin tones: fair skin, with pink overtones, which he calls "cold-toned skin," and skin with a yellow tone to it, such as olive skin, which he calls "warm-toned." (And yes, skin tone can change according to the season.) If your skin is cold-toned, you should choose a shade of cheek color in the pink-to-purple range. If it's warm-toned, a brownish, peach, or taupe cheek color will look best. Most women can get away with wearing more than one color of rouge or blusher. A good time to change your cheek color is summer, when you're tan, or after you've just done some outdoor sport and have one of those healthy pink glows we've all heard so much about. In any case, you'll certainly want to vary it according to your mood and the occasion. François offers a very soothing suggestion: after you've applied your basic cheek color, add a very light pink color. "Only pink," he says, "can *really* warm up the skin." Whatever color rouge or blush-on you select should emphasize rather than be at odds with your natural skin tone. (And if something shouldn't be at odds with something else, then it should be even with it, right?)

## EYECOLOR PENCILS

These are just soft crayons made of waxes, pigments, and oils. I have half a dozen of them in different subtle colors. You can use them both as liners and as shadows for the eyes.

### How to Use Them

Sharpen the pencil to a blunt point, then line your eyes by drawing a thin, continuous line just above the lashes, and beneath the lashes on the lower lid. Now blend the line by smudging it with your finger. This blending process is essential, because what you want to do is create a shadowy line, not a hard, definite one. Lining the eyes both above and below makes the lashes appear thicker and creates a sultry effect suited to those daydreams that are often the little props of our personalities. You can also use the eyecolor pencil to shade the eyelid.

### How to Choose Them

It's important that you select a pencil with the right texture for your skin type. If the pencil is too hard, it's

Make up by
François Ilasehen...

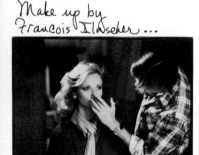

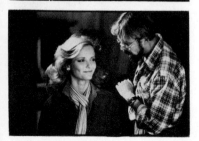

going to pull on your eyelid and may even damage the delicate skin there; if it's too soft and greasy, it may run, and before you know it you'll be embarrassed at finding the color on other parts of your face. I prefer muted colors for lining my eyes: brown, mauve, navy, and charcoal gray, which create a shadow—not a distinct color—on the eyelid. These colors go well with all eye colors and all skin tones. My guru François says that to make the eyes stand out, the frame of liner around them should be darker than the irises and that the darker your eyes are, the darker the frames should be. Brown-eyed women, then, should line their eyes with a very dark black, blue, purple, or brown pencil, and women with light blue eyes should use a blue or gray or brown.

Eyeliner also comes in a cake form, which you can just brush on with water. This type of liner can create an extremely soft look if you carefully wet the brush, run it over the cake, then brush the liner as close to the base of the lashes as possible, using your finger to smudge before the ink dries.

## EYE SHADOW

And God created eye shadow . . . to emphasize the color of your eyes. I believe in keeping it really simple —sticking to one or two shades. Your eyelid isn't a canvas for an abstract expressionist painting, so why pile on a huge eruption of colors that will only call so much attention to your eye shadow that nobody will even notice the shape and color of your eyes?

### How to Choose It

Eyeshadow is available in creams, liquids, and creamy, pressed powders. The creams and liquids blend well with the eyelid but might crease with time. Eyeshadows differ markedly in consistency; also, once on, they may look quite different from how they looked in that fancy container—so, again, sample *before* you buy.

Never use a shadow that matches either the color of your eyes or the outfit you're wearing. If you have green eyes and wear a bright green shadow, it's going to be hard to see the true color of your eyes. According to François, whose business it is to know everyone's facial weaknesses, the color of shadow that is most flattering to you is the one *opposite* to your eye color on the color spectrum. The opposite, or contradictory, or complementary color of blue, for example, is

for Cover Girl.
My New York Family

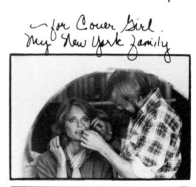

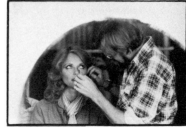

yellow, brown, or orange, and François often uses a gold, almost orange shadow on blue eyes. By the same token, brown eyes look great with gray or purple shadow, and green or hazel eyes with purple or pink.

If you take the trouble to examine the iris of your eye closely in a hand mirror, you won't see just one color there, but many—specks of brown, gold, gray, mauve. Select one of these secondary colors and use it as a guide. Eyeshadow was meant to live up to its name, to create a shadow rather than an actual color on your lid. The neutral shades like brown, gray, and mauve, come in a wide variety of colors: gray, for instance, can be gray-mauve, pale silver gray, green-gray, blue-gray, or charcoal gray. And brown can be russet, coppery, or gray-brown.

## MASCARA

Mascara is one of the cosmetics that can make the most difference in how you look. It not only emphasizes but deepens the eyes, giving them a dark, expressive quality. I brush-pat on a light coat for daytime and apply extra coats for evening.

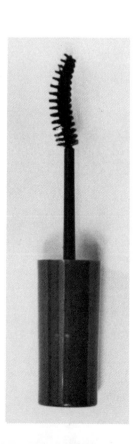

### How to Use It

The secret of applying mascara is to brush on a thin coat, from the base of your lashes to the tip, and let it dry completely. Don't "dump" the wand into the applicator, it'll only make it wet and gooey—and be sure it isn't loaded with gobs of mascara that will end up under your eyes. I really prefer a slightly older mascara, because the liquid inside is drier and easier to handle. If you're applying several coats, wait till each one dries before putting on the next. After your mascara is all dry, separate the lashes with a small brush —a child's toothbrush is perfect for this—unless you want your lashes clumped together in artificial-looking, artery-hardening spikes. That look went out of the window with Mary Poppins.

### How to Choose It

A good mascara will go on smoothly and won't leave little flakes on your lashes, or clump them together, or go gallivanting to other parts of the eye area. It will come off easily, too. The most modern type is the wand and tube which allows them quantity and consistency control, but some women like the old-fashioned cake and brush. The most natural-looking color is black, or dark brown for a slightly softer look. The colored mascaras can be too obvious and anyway don't add enough depth to the eye. One thing: you have to be prepared to buy a new mascara every six months, because older ones can carry infection-forming bacteria.

## EYEBROW PENCIL

Don't look startled when I say that very few women *need* an eyebrow pencil. If you've tweezed your eyebrows into an attractive shape, they shouldn't have to be darkened with any pencil. The experts feel that your brows should be a shade lighter than your hair color, and they recommend bleaching brows that are so dark they overpower face and eyes. I seldom use the pencil. I have pale eyebrows, and occasionally I feather a few light lines into them. If your eyebrows are sparse, buy a soft-colored pencil (never a black one), or a powder, or consider having your brows tweezed by a professional. But easy-does-it, don't tweeze those eyebrows out of existence. And never extend your eyebrow line out toward your temple, Fu-Manchu style, unless you're planning to audition for a part in a Far Eastern flick.

## LIPSTICK AND LIP GLOSS

You may think that this is odd coming from a professional model *but:* I hardly ever wear lipstick. Most of the lipstick in my cosmetic kit I use for model assignments only. I use just a touch of natural or pink lipgloss to make my lips shiny and moist and to balance out the colors on my face. A lot of lipstick can look pretty snazzy but you run the risk of overemphasizing your mouth, making it look hard, or painted like a clown's (though probably not as friendly).

### How to Use Them

Apply lip color with a lipstick brush, and you can control the density of the color and where it goes—also, the lip color stays on longer. Then blend into your lips. And buy the small, squarish hardibrush, made especially with lipstick in mind. When you smear on lipstick or gloss with a tube or with your finger, you inevitably find it's escaped, gotten outside the contours of your lips. In fact, it's usually all over your fingers, and this is one case where you *don't* want to let your fingers do the talking!

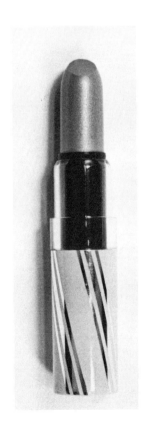

### How to Choose Them

Lip color should blend with your skin tone. And unlike eye color and cheek color, it should take its cue partly from the colors you are wearing. Who would ever want to wear mauve or orange lipstick with a bright red blouse? Most women can wear several different shades of lip color. Almost anyone can wear a clear red in a modern sheer lipstick or gloss. Fair-skinned women look good in pink-toned lip colors; women with sallow skin can wear colors in the peach-to-brown range. But always remember, what looks good in the tube or on someone else might not look so good on you, because your skin chemistry changes the color of the lipstick once it's on your lips.

## HIGHLIGHTING CREAMS

They're great fun for evening: they emphasize your bones and add some excitement to your face. I apply a pearly white, almost translucent cream to my cheekbones and to the bone beneath my eyebrows. Sometimes I use a mauve, iridescent cream blended right into my skin so I don't get that garish, clown-like effect. Highlighters are available in pencil and in cream and liquid.

## THREE TIME-SAVING MAKEUP LOOKS

Once you've selected cosmetics in the colors and textures that become you and, most important, learned how to get the most out of them and make them work for you, the actual application should take only a few minutes. Here are three sure-fire step-by-step formulas for applying makeup. Please follow my instructions in detail.

### C.T.'s 10-Minute Natural Makeup Look

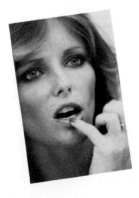

1. After you have your moisturizer on, apply a base lightly to your face and neck with your fingertips.
2. Apply an eyeliner just above your upper lashes and below your lower lashes with eyeliner pencil in a soft, muted shade. Blend with your fingertip.
3. Apply one light coat of mascara and let it dry.
4. Apply a cream or liquid cheek color to your cheekbones and blend out toward your temples.
5. Apply a natural or pale lipstick or gloss. Before you leave the house, check your makeup in natural light from the window to make sure your base is on

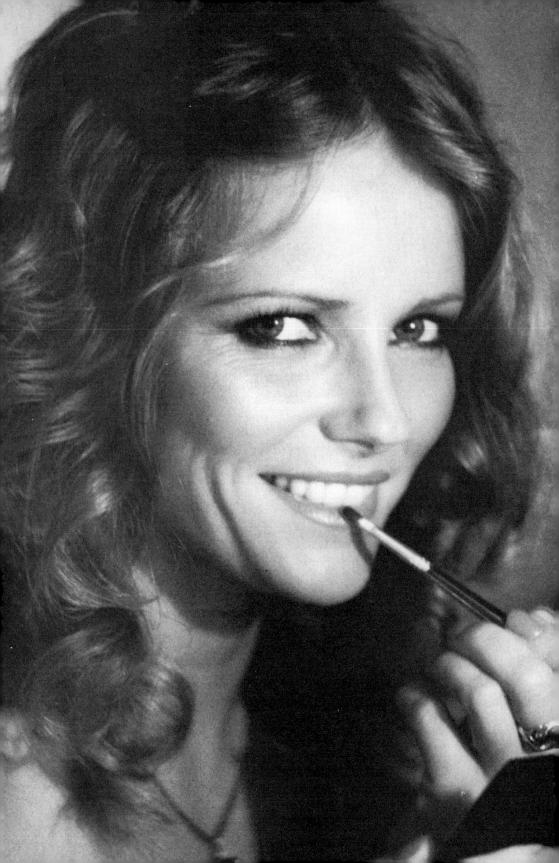

evenly and the colors you've applied have blended well. This subtle, no-makeup look not only adds a little color to your face, but heightens your natural coloring.

### C.T.'s 15-Minute Evening Makeup Look

1. Apply the base as in the 10-minute makeup look. Don't pile on twice as much just because the sun's gone down. Let the sun be always on your cheeks, let your skin show through.

2. Line your eyes with a dark-colored pencil, above the lash line and below the lower lashes.

3. Apply a pressed powder eyeshadow from your eyelashes to beneath your eyebrow. Now shade your eyelid, from corner to corner, with a darker shadow (brown, gray, mauve). You may want to extend the shadow beyond the corner of your eye and blend it into the skin. Blend with a brush or your fingertip, so no line of the powder can be seen. ("The art that conceals art"—remember?)

4. Apply one coat of mascara and let it dry. Then apply another coat.

5. Apply a powdered blusher with a large sable brush, and blend thoroughly.

6. Apply a colored lip gloss or a sheer lipstick.

7. Dust with a translucent powder before you leave the house.

### C.T.'s 20-Minute Makeup for Glamorous Nights

1. Apply the makeup base as above.

2. Apply eyeshadow as in the 15-minute makeup exercise, possibly a tad more.

3. Add a bit of gold eyeshadow or a shimmery copper or silver to the middle of your eyelid, lightly around the eye.

4. Apply eyeliner as in 15-minute makeup exercise, using a deep shade of blue or a dark charcoal.

5. Apply two or three coats of mascara. Let each coat dry completely before you apply the next—separating the lashes with a brush if necessary. Be sure to get every lash—the ones at the corner of the eye are important, too.

6. Apply a powdered blusher in a couple of shades; use the more intense color for night lighting.

7. Add just a touch of magenta or white highlighting cream to your eyebone and cheekbone and blend thoroughly. This is the step that really gives you a romantic evening look!

8. Now apply a bright shade of lipstick (clear red, pink, mauve, or coral). Add a clear lip gloss.

9. Dust your whole face with translucent powder.

## MAKEUP TECHNIQUES FOR EXTRA GLAMOUR

For the purest, richest glamour—glamour to spare, glamour to bathe in—try the following (but not all of them at once, please—one or two at a time should do the trick).

1. Line the inside of your eye, just above the lashes, with a deep-colored pencil—navy blue, deep purple. This will make the color and shape of your eyes stand out like headlights.

2. If you have any clothes that are electric blue, bright green, or magenta, add a *dot* of the same color eyeshadow to the middle of your eyelid or the corner of your eye, and blend slightly.

3. Shade the center of your lower lip with a deeper color.

4. Add a touch of color glow liquid in pink, mauve, gold, or bronze to your usual base.

5. Instead of ordinary translucent powder, use a fine gold or silver powder to dust your face.

When you apply makeup, if possible use a mirror lighted from both sides. Light coming from above, or from one side only, is going to illuminate only one side of your face, and as a result you may make the mistake of applying more makeup to one half than the other.

The key thing to remember about night makeup: don't put it on thicker and darker so that nothing of your real face shines through the cracks and you can't find your way back to it. It's the bits of sparkle that make the difference here.

## OUTWITTING YOUR FLAWS

Some say that makeup can successfully conceal flaws. Sorry but I just don't believe that the flaws in a person's face can be blotted out by cosmetics. (*Modified*, yes.) If you opt for elaborate shading to "fix" a crooked nose, or cover your eyes with tons of shadow in the forlorn hope of changing their shape, or line your lips with a vivid pencil trying to change their natural curve, take my word for it—I've been there—you'll only succeed in making yourself—and everyone else! —*more* conscious of the so-called flaw.

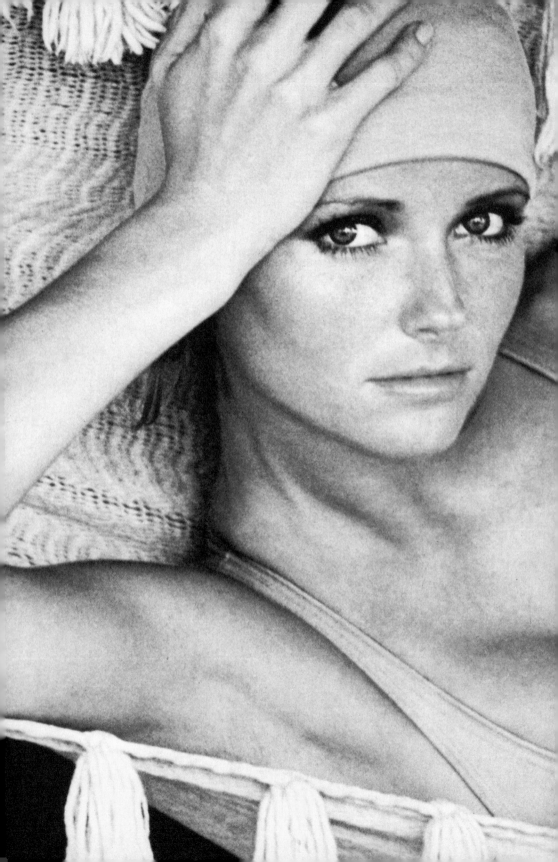

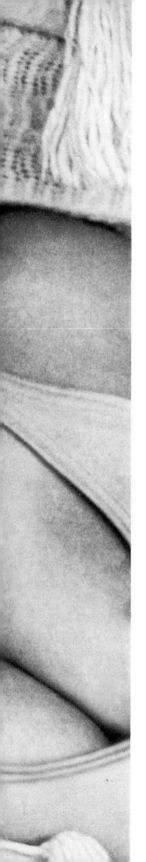

Moreover, you will probably botch the job, and make your skin look all muddy or uneven. I can't say it often enough, here goes: you don't want people to notice your makeup, you want them to notice your face! I confess to having shaded the sides of my nose with brown powder to make it look "stronger" in a photograph, but I've done this in the line of "duty": little sculpting tricks that work for the camera—helping you to create the kind of look you want that feature to have in the final photograph—in real life register loud and clear (and thick) as makeup. I've noticed that women tend to single out a feature on their face and judge it *too* harshly. Often the feature they happen to dislike is not a "flaw," it's just unusual or different (it may even add something to their face). If you think your face has a "flaw," try looking at it in a less trivial and self-conscious light, and from a new perspective —in combination with your other features.

For those who do decide to try a little trick to improve a feature, here's a list of some simple makeup techniques of mine which really do work and better yet, don't involve a great deal of shading, sketching, or contouring. Just keep in mind that dark shading makes an area recede while light shading emphasizes it.

### Concealing Dark Shadows Beneath the Eyes

The best shadow-concealing technique I know is also the simplest: apply a light coat of your usual makeup base to the dark area—if you use a lighter concealing stick, make sure you use it subtly, and blend carefully so you don't have an obvious white area. You have to realize that it's impossible to conceal any shadow completely. Lining your eyes beneath the lower lashes with a gray, brown, or steel-dark blue eye pencil, will deflect attention from the circle.

### Small Eyes

To make your eyes look bigger, begin your liner in the middle of the upper lid and extend it to the outside corner, and repeat this process below the lower lashes. (The line should be thin and subtle.) Curl your lashes with an eyelash curler. Apply mascara very sparingly; use a smoky shadow in the crease on the lid. Be extra-careful not to load down your eyes with the dead, dead weight of too much makeup, which will hide and annihilate them.

### Wide-Set Eyes

If you want to bring them a bit closer together, start your shadow at the corner by your nose and extend it along the crease. Apply mascara most heavily to the lashes closest to your nose. Don't over-emphasize the part of your eyebrow closest to the nose, and don't extend the browline in that direction—leave the eyebrows natural!

### Close-Set Eyes

To make close-set eyes look further apart, accent the outer corners by beginning your shadow at the middle of the lid and extending it past the corner of the eye. Now blend. Apply several coats of mascara to the lashes closest to the outside corner of the eye.

### A Wide Forehead

I have one, and I minimize it by shading along the hairline (both sides and top).

### A Wide Jawline

If your jawline is too wide or "strong," you can minimize it by brushing both sides of your jaw with blush-on and then blending.

### A Narrow Jawline

To emphasize your jawline, brush it with a light powder.

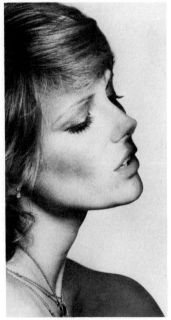

### Imperfect Lips

A line drawn around the lips with a pencil can make you look iron-hard. If you do use a pencil, select one that's almost the same color as your lips—and blend carefully so you can't see a line when you're finished. The color of the lipstick or gloss you choose can do a lot for the shape of your lips. If your mouth is wide, use a light, sheer gloss or lipstick, and apply sparingly. Don't emphasize the outer edges of your lips. If they're thin, stay away from frosted shades of lipstick. (Come to think of it, everyone should avoid frosted shades of lipstick.) And too much lipstick, unless it's applied with great skill, can make thin lips look even thinner.

### Hidden Cheekbones

If your cheekbones aren't high or prominent enough to suit you, put an accent above the cheekbone with a light highlighting cream, and blend well, then place your blush or rouge just below the bone and extend it out toward the temple.

### Blemishes

Don't try to hide a blemish—you'll only arouse suspicion. Just apply your regular makeup base, and dab a little extra on the blemish, along with the tiniest bit of concealing stick or special blemish cream. I've found that powder helps dry up a blemish faster than any liquid base does. Be very careful when you brush the powder on that you don't brush away the base and the concealer.

### Sallow, Pale, or Ruddy Skin

If your skin is an unhealthy color, it's trying to tell you something—like go get some fresh air and exercise! You can liven up pale or sallow skin another, less strenuous way. Use a pink-tinted color-glow foundation instead of your usual base, or brush a neutral shade of blusher on the tip of your chin, forehead, and cheekbones. If you're sunburned, or if your skin is on the ruddy side, use an ivory-colored base over an aqua or green-tinted liquid foundation to neutralize your skin tone.

## MAKING THE MOST OF YOUR MAKEUP

### Keeping Makeup Where It Belongs

If your lipstick has a tendency to disappear or run, apply a light base coat of foundation before you add any lip color. If your eye makeup also tends to slip away or crease on your lid, apply a base coat of foundation and a bit of powder to your eyelids as well. Some cosmetics companies sell a neutral eyelid foundation especially designed to provide a secure base for eye color. Brushing a little translucent powder over your lashes will help keep the mascara in place and make your lashes look thicker.

### Refreshing Tired Makeup

If your makeup gets "tired," as it is apt to during a night on the town, you can refresh it with minimal effort and equipment. What I do is blot my base with a damp tissue or cloth to remove some of the shine, then moisten a Q-tip and dab away any specks of mascara or eyeshadow that have landed beneath my eyes; then I freshen the eyeshadow and blush-on, brighten my eyes with eyedrops, add a touch of extra lip gloss, and *presto magico!* I feel and look like new. Unless you have world enough and time, taking all your makeup off and putting it on again can leave your eyes and face red from all the rubbing and pulling. Besides, makeup always looks better when it's had a chance to settle and soak in.

### Achieving with the Bare-Minimum Look

If I'm off to the beach or tennis courts and want to add some shine to my face without going to all the trouble of putting on actual makeup, I just apply a sunscreen and a shiny lip protection stick.

### Treating Yourself to the Tea-Bag Treatment

If you've over-indulged yourself, or are under a great deal of stress, with the usual accompaniment of sleepless nights, telltale sacks and bags will begin to make an appearance under your eyes. This is, as the Austrians like to say, "serious but not hopeless" (rather than "hopeless but not serious," which the Germans like to say).

I have a good home remedy for the "Puffs." I lie down, put my feet up, and cover my eyes with wet tea bags (any brand will do). The tannic acid in the tea acts as an astringent, has a soothing effect on the eyes, and reduces the swelling. The tea-bag treatment also calms me down, helps me get back onto myself and away from whatever generated those nasty puffs in the first place. (The alternative is getting your personality to conform to the puffs, and I don't think you want to do that.)

### Battling the Fluorescent Lights

Many offices and public places are guilty of the bad taste of having fluorescent lighting that drains the color from people's faces and makes them look sickly, if not actually moribund. If you have to spend a lot of time under such lights, use warm colors in cosmetics —red, orange, and golden tones (pinks are out because, surprisingly, they contain blues, as do certain wines and mauves). Experiment with using a foundation in a deeper shade than usual. Also, apply your makeup under a—shudder!—fluorescent light, so you'll know just how it's going to look.

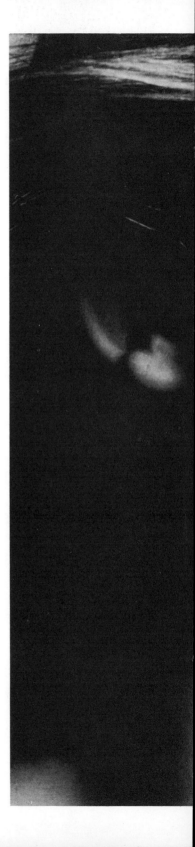

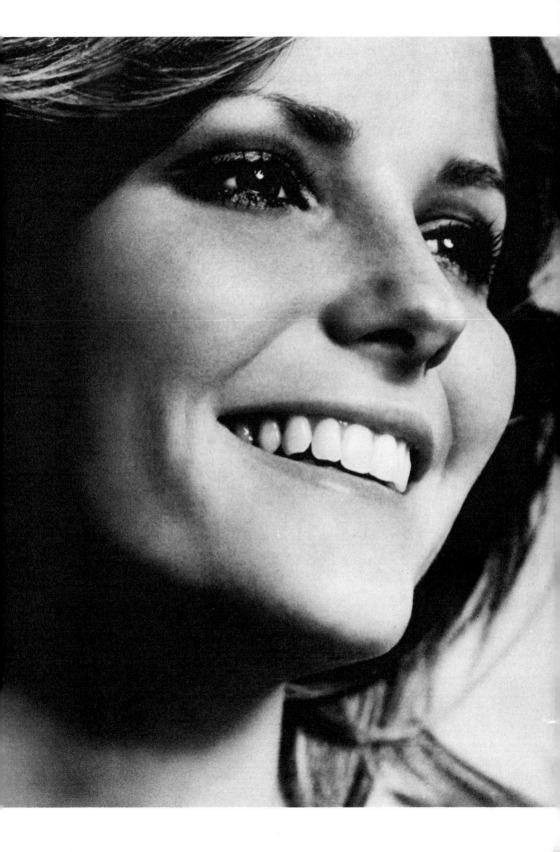

### Giving Yourself the Deep Frost

One of the best ways to use a frosted shade of eyeshadow, lipstick, or cheek color is to use it *underneath* a matte shade. This disposition will give the matte some depth and that longed-for sparkle.

## MISTAKES PEOPLE MAKE WITH MAKEUP

### Not Blending or Checking

The single biggest mistake you can make with makeup is not blending it into your skin. The result is hard lines and great gobs of color that don't look like they belong on your face. Always take that extra second or two to smudge your eyeliner with your fingertip and blend your makeup base, cheek color, and eyeshadow. Also, check your makeup in different kinds of lighting to make sure it still looks natural.

### Piling It on Under Glass

Don't put extra makeup on your eyes just because you happen to wear glasses. Make up your eyes as subtly as you do the rest of your face. Overdoing it won't make your glasses disappear or your eyes stand out more.

### Over-tweezing Eyebrows

Once upon a time, an over-eager makeup artist tweezed my eyebrows down to a two-hairline. "You'll thank me for this," he said. (He might better have said, "Years from now when you write about this, and you will, be kind.") But when I saw my no-eyebrow look in the mirror, I burst into tears for the first time since I hit the scales at 150. Eyebrows should neither dominate your face nor be totally invisible. The danger of over-tweezing for a long period of time is that the hairs may never grow back. To keep the shape of your eyebrows natural, tweeze only underneath and neaten up the middle between the brows. And pull in the direction the hair grows; this may hurt a little, so you'll want to use a cream, both before and after.

### Not Removing Makeup Before Turning in

We all get lazy, but don't worry, we pay for it. Go to bed with your eyes loaded down with shadow and mascara and your skin covered with blusher and base, and you'll wake up looking like the sergeant's mess (eye makeup smeared on cheeks, and puffy swollen eyes, and skin that never even got a chance to breathe).

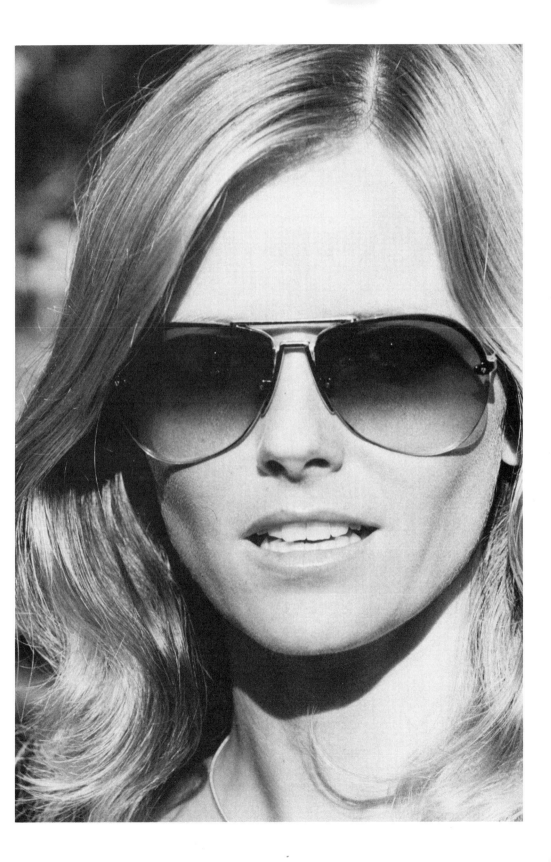

### Applying Bilious Blue and
### Green Gage Eyeshadow

These outdated bright shades will completely mask the color of your eyes. If you can't bring yourself to toss your blue and green shadows in the wastepaper basket, where they belong, try combining them with charcoal grays or browns, which will at least tone them down, if not neutralize them.

### Not Concentrating

When you put on your makeup, concentrate! Forget how late you are for work or what's for breakfast. If your mind is wandering, you may mistakenly use a rouge-covered fingertip to blend your eyeshadow, or smear your lipstick, or brush on your blusher where it doesn't belong. Work carefully: wash or wipe your hands when necessary, use the right tools, do yourself up, do yourself proud. Outdo yourself.

### Making Like "The Dragon Lady"

Never draw a slanted line past the corner of your eyes with eyeliner—it will make you look bestial and predatory. It's okay to extend the liner slightly beyond the corner of your eye, but be sure to smudge the line with your finger so there's only a slight shadow.

### Experimenting at the Next-to-Last Minute

Get to know your face and makeup before the crucial moment comes when you have to put the two together for the outside world. Your spare time is the time to fool around with new makeup techniques and products. If you do botch your makeup before an important occasion, don't fall apart and try to repair the mistake by applying even more makeup. Just go back to your tried-and-true basic ways.

There's no excuse in this day and age for not looking your best. As the great French writer Colette wrote in *Earthly Paradise:* "Where are those rouges of yesteryear, with their harsh red currant tints, those ungrateful whites, those Virgin Mary blues? We now have a range of tints at our disposal that would go to the head of a painter." Right on!

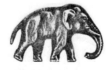

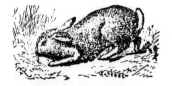

# 7

## Saving Your Own Skin

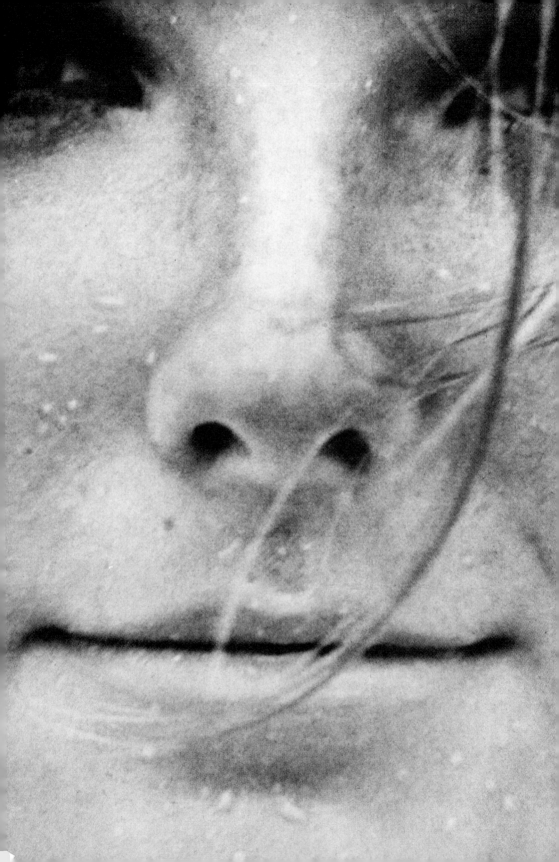

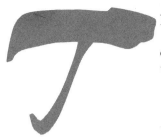

The skin is the only organ we possess that's ever on public display. Among other things, this miraculous envelope regulates body temperature and employs its network of delicate nerves as sentinels for both pleasure and pain. As such, skin can tell us what's happening inside and outside our bodies. It reflects our diet, the amount of exercise we get, our health habits (good and bad), our age, hormonal balance, heredity—and—not least of all—emotional state. In fact, it's the multiplicity of factors influencing the way our skin looks that makes it disobedient to our little tricks and most ardent ministrations. No wonder few of us find ourselves with the skin we would ideally like to have—soft, even-toned, blemish-free, aglow with the color of life. (Some of us aren't very comfortable in our own skins—the French have a wonderful way of expressing this: *On n'est pas bien dans sa peau*," they say. But that's another story.)

Every woman wants a beautiful complexion, but to achieve it she must be prepared to work. She may be more inclined to do so if she recalls that it is her skin that stands between her and the world.

Skin may not be deep, but it *is* sensitive; it needs to be nourished, stimulated, and protected. The first step is to analyze your skin type. Sift through the wealth of information available about skin care, appropriating the facts that apply to you and discarding the others. Then experiment intelligently with the many skin products on the market.

How much *do* you know about your own skin? Mark the following ten statements "true" or "false," and you'll have some idea.

■ *Creams and moisturizers prevent wrinkles.*

■ *Damage to the epidermis caused by excessive sunbathing eventually heals.*

■ *Baby oil helps protect your skin from the sun.*

■ *A woman's skin can be classified as oily, dry, or "normal." More than fifty percent of the female population has "normal" skin.*

■ *Women with oily skin should not use moisturizers.*

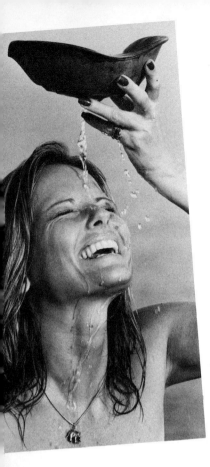

- *There is basically no difference between an astringent and a freshening lotion.*

- *Acne is not affected by diet.*

- *"Blackheads" are a sign that you are not washing your face enough.*

- *The benefits of a skin masque are primarily psychological.*

- *You should bathe or shower at least once a day.*

Every single one of the above statements is false. Now let's find out why.

## THE IMPORTANCE OF SKIN CARE

When I was a formless teenager (or, in the poet Robert Lowell's beautiful phrase, "back in my shaggy throwaway of adolescence"), even when I didn't have actual blemishes, my skin was dry and flaky. As you know by now, I sweetened puberty for myself by means of all kinds of unjust desserts and junk food. It was no big shock to me when I put on weight; what *was* shocking was that the bad food was damaging my skin as well as my figure.

I never really bothered much about my skin. I would spend an entire day in the photographer's studio, piling on acres of makeup, and then go right out to dinner with friends, after which, if it was a typical evening, I'd be far too tired to wash off all the foundation, powder, rouge, etcetera. I'd just fall into bed grateful for the pillow's soft, obliterating white. I would give my face a thorough cleaning once a day only, when I took my morning shower, and I would use the same strong soap on it as I did on the rest of my body. Afterwards, my face would feel taut, dry, and stretched, and I thought that this was exactly how it *should* feel and that I didn't need to use a drop of moisturizer. What arrogance! What ignorance! No wonder my skin was dry!!

Sometimes at a party I would notice that my all-day mascara had slipped down beneath my eyes. I'd then try removing the black specks by dabbing at them indiscriminately with a soapy Kleenex; and after this, I wouldn't even bother to rinse the drying soap away. In the years that have passed since then, I have learned that skin is far more vulnerable than ever I imagined —particularly the skin under the eyes.

I never had acne—thank God, because a mere pimple was enough to throw me off balance. When I began posing for magazine covers, I discovered how photographers' close-up lenses and bright lights heartlessly reveal flaws in even the most perfect complexions. "Flaws," I call them—well, I always loved a euphemism. Joseph Conrad called them "grogblossoms" (at least in his great novel, *Youth*, he did). But of course your classmates always called them pimples or, worse, "zits." The photographers assured me that they could retouch the blemishes, and sure enough, they had all been airbrushed away by the final photographic print. However, it was beyond any photographer's power to make them disappear from my face. It never occurred to me that my terrible diet and the lack of attention I was giving my skin (negligence may be a more honest description) had much of anything to do with these flaws. I sort of assumed that the people with forever clear skin were just lucky and that the rest of us, in varying degrees, weren't. It was easy to lay it all on fate, and go back to grimly covering my face with makeup and hoping the spots would fade away.

One day a friend, another model, took me aside and gently—kindly—suggested I see a cosmetician. He in turn gave me special products and worked up a skin-cleaning routine for me to practice at home. Loaded down with special soaps and multicolored lotions, and resenting the expense of the visit, I went sulking back to my apartment. But for the first time in my life I began to give my skin the attention it needed and deserved. Nobody was more surprised than I was when it began to clear. From having been worked on so consistently, my face at first was very dry, but little by little the texture improved and the blemishes disappeared. My whole face felt softer and smoother. It was like a grace.

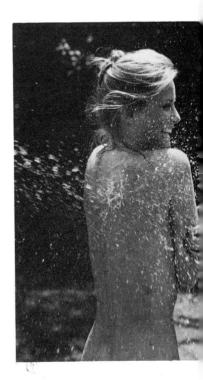

I remember how, soon after this, I caught sight of my reflection in a store window and doubled back to take a second look. I couldn't believe that this lucky stranger with the clear skin was me. It was about this time that I went on the diet to which I owe my dramatic weight loss. At last I was on the verge of being on good physical terms with myself. Talk about castles in the sky!

Blemished skin, oily skin, dry skin, "muddy" skin with unhealthy-looking shadows, diddy-daddied skin,

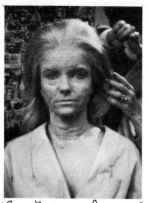

and sallow skin all respond very positively to the following *natural* practices:

■ *Proper cleansing, toning, and moisturizing with products designed for your type of skin.*

■ *Treatment of blemishes—with professional help when necessary.*

■ *Deep-cleansing facials.*

■ *Good diet, exercise, and plenty of rest.*

■ *Regulated exposure to the sun.*

But first things first.

## DIAGNOSING YOUR SKIN TYPE

This may be more difficult than it sounds, because you can't permanently "typecast" your skin. Oily skin, for example, may become drier in winter when it's exposed to blasts of both central heating and cold air, and even oilier in summer. When I was working in Africa on my ABC-TV special, my ordinarily dry skin got drier and drier. Stress, a change of environment, changes in hormone levels, a new diet, pregnancy, use of medication, menopause, and the whole process of aging (which is, alas, often quite independent of the calendar), can transform your skin for better or worse —it's all something of a lottery, at the mercy of more things than even dermatologists can fathom. I know of practically no one over the age of twelve who has skin that is never tarnished by blemishes, dry flakes, or traces of oil. If your skin looks "normal" most of the time, it's got to be because you are successfully protecting it and keeping it properly nourished.

Now: What skin type *are* you?

*Dry skin* usually feels "tight" or "taut" for hours after you've washed it. It's also marked by flakes, causing makeup to congeal in the dry areas—to the extent that, if your skin is very dry, it may almost hurt when you smile. (But don't not smile!) Dry skin is usually marked by superficial lines as well. It chaps quickly and may even "crack" in cold weather, and in the sun it burns, baby, burns. On the bright side, it's often so finely textured that you can't even see the pores.

*Oily skin* generally takes on a greasy shine shortly after being washed; when you touch it with your fin-

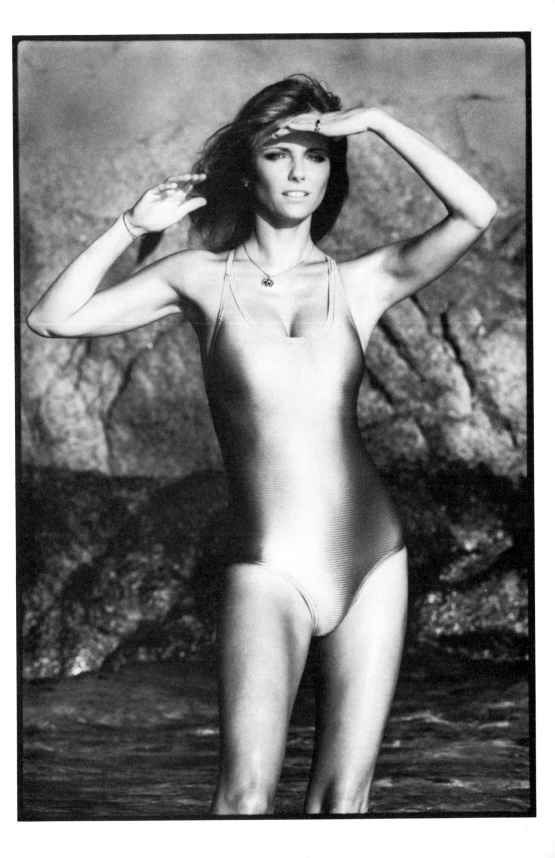

gers, it feels all "slick." It also absorbs makeup, sometimes even changing the color of it. Blackheads, whiteheads, and pimples seem to gravitate to oily skin with its enlarged pores. Oily skin can be dull and, above all, flaky (which is great if you're a piecrust but not so great if you're a human). Surprisingly, oily skin is often mistaken for dry skin, and thus incorrectly treated. The flakes, especially if they're accompanied by raised red spots, are sometimes caused by an inflammation called "seborrheic dermatitis." (This condition calls for a dermatologist and plenty of cortisone cream.) A plus factor is that, because oily skin by definition provides its own lubrication, it's not so susceptible to developing fine lines.

*Combination skin* is just that: oily and dry, or normal in some areas and dry or oily in others. The really oily areas are the nose, forehead and chin.

## CLEANSING, TONING, AND MOISTURIZING (OR C.T.'S GUARANTEED C-T-M REGIMEN)

Whatever skin type you have must be cleansed, toned, and moisturized daily. This routine will vary slightly according to skin type, and will take only a few minutes a day. If your skin is still too dry and lifeless, or too oily, or too *anything*, the products you're using are the wrong ones for you—or else your skin has done a number and changed. Most skins, however, will respond to careful handling. Just don't expect the major changes to occur overnight! If you don't have confidence in your own ability to diagnose your skin type or to find the right products, pay a visit to a cosmetician, as I did. The initial investment may be irritatingly high, but you'll ultimately save money you'd otherwise waste on a lot of probably useless experiments with the wrong products.

### Cleansing

*Dry Skin.* Dry skin should be cleansed in the morning to remove the impurities it's accumulated during sleep, and at night to remove those it's accumulated during the day. Many women with dry skin are afraid that cleansing their faces with soap and water will just dry them out more. A mild soap, dermatologists agree, is the best emulsifier of dirt and oil; water is what moisturizes the skin from within and should not be avoided at any cost. Dry-skinned women must be especially careful about choosing the right soap, such as superfatted soap containing olive oil, or a fine oatmeal soap. Transparent soaps with a glycerin base should be avoided, as they may contain drying alcohol and in any case aren't as gentle as they're reputed to be. Like many other women with delicate skin, I prefer to use a special cleansing lotion. Most of these lotions contain a very mild soap (make sure yours doesn't contain alcohol). Some cleansing agents require rinsing with lukewarm water. To avoid irritation, don't wash your face just before you go outside in winter.

*How to Wash.* Massage the soap or cleansing lotion into your skin with circular motions of your fingertips. The drier and more delicate your skin is, the more gently you should massage.

*Oily Skin.* Oily skin needs to be washed more often than dry skin—as much as three or four times a day. The best cleanser is a soap containing a small quantity of sulphur, alcohol, or salicylic acid. People with very oily or blemish-prone skin often prefer a cleansing grain, which is a soap composed of tiny, abrasive particles that are very effective in unclogging oily pores. There are also some cleansing lotions on the market that are especially geared to oily skin. Rinse your face thoroughly—some cosmeticians recommend twenty to thirty splashes of water (warm, not hot, as hot water may stimulate oil flow instead of stanching it).

*Combination Skin.* The cleansing agent you use should depend, naturally, on your particular combination. Many cleansing lotions and soaps were concocted for normal or oily skin, and they might just be your best bet. A cleansing grain, or epidermabrading agent, you'll probably want to save mostly for oily areas.

## Toning

A toning lotion will rid your skin of the impurities that are left after you've worked with a cleansing agent or water; it stimulates circulation in your skin, trims the top layer of cells, and tightens your pores (temporarily).

*Dry Skin.* Dry skin should be toned with a mild skin-freshening lotion that does *not* contain alcohol. Apply with a cotton pad.

*Oily Skin.* Oily skin is best toned with an astringent lotion with a slight alcohol base. If this proves too harsh, switch to a freshening lotion with no alcohol whatsoever. Wipe the astringent onto the skin firmly with a cotton pad.

*Combination Skin.* Combination skin can be well served by two toners—one without alcohol for the dry areas, and one with alcohol for the oily T-zone. If you use only one toner, go the teetotalling way: no alcohol!

## Moisturizing

Creams and moisturizers don't actually add moisture to your skin; what they do is seal in the skin's natural water so it won't evaporate. They also help the skin retain the oils produced by the skin glands. They lubricate the skin and though they can't prevent wrinkles, they fill in tiny lines and soften the edges; and finally they form a film protecting the skin from harsh pollutants and inclement weather.

*Dry Skin.* Dry skin all but cries out for a moisturizer. Make it a point to apply a light-textured moisturizer once or twice during the day, and a heavier cream at night.

*Oily Skin.* To moisturize or not to moisturize: that is the question for cosmeticians. I believe that every skin should be moisturized, if only for protective purposes. If your skin is oily, select your moisturizer with great care—a heavy, oily moisturizer may further block your pores and cause unsightly flare-ups. Some cosmetics companies feature lotions that blot the oil while they soften the skin and protect it from the environment. I certainly don't advise heavy night creams for oily skin.

*Combination Skin.* This type of skin needs a little extra attention. The dry areas may have to be moisturized more often and with a different product from the one you use on oily areas.

*Applying Moisturizer.* No matter what type of skin you have, applying too much moisturizer is as bad as applying none at all. There is only so much that even a moisturizer can do, so don't go putting on thick layers in the mistaken belief that "more is better." Tiny dabs, applied with a circular motion, will blend the moisturizer more evenly into your skin.

*Moisturizing Your Eyes.* The area around the eyes has no oil glands and should therefore definitely be moisturized. I dab a special eye cream around my eyes each night—very carefully, so the cream doesn't ooze into my eyes while I'm sleeping (I don't want to wake up with puffy lids). Don't rub or pull on the very delicate skin around the eyes—wrinkles, sags, and long-term stretches are lying in wait for you.

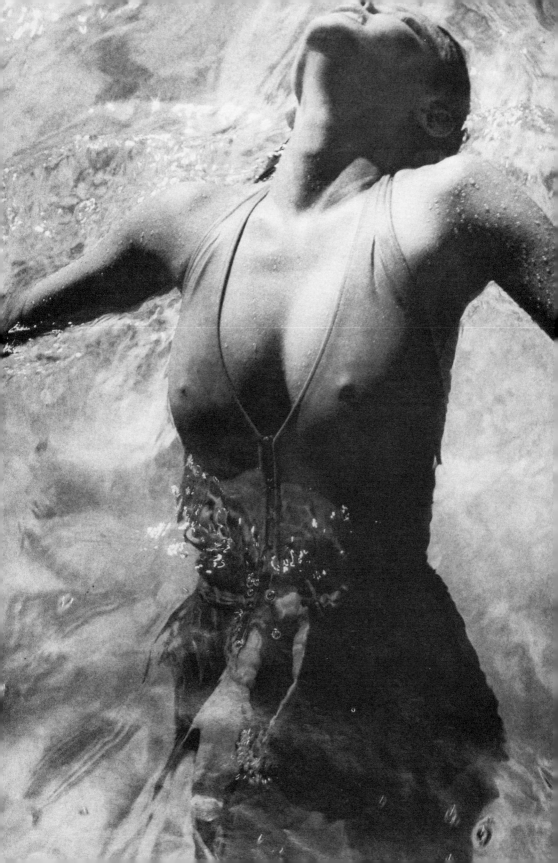

# THE ORIGIN OF ACNE—
# AND SOME NEW HOPE

Acne (I even hate the *sound* of the word) is the result of the malfunctioning of the thousands of oil glands near the hair follicles, which produce too much oil or "sebum." Oil normally escapes through pores; in acne-prone skin, however, the cells that line the oil ducts build up, stick together, and block the flow of excess oil. The trapped oil then forms a microscopic whitehead below the surface of the skin, where the bacteria in the pores can act on it. When this plug of oil, bacteria, and cells pushes its way to the surface of the skin, it oxidizes in the air and turns black. It's a common belief that "blackheads" are caused by inadequate cleansing, but this just isn't so—they represent a mild form of acne, beginning below the skin surface. Luckily, you can squeeze them out fairly easily or sometimes simply wash them off. If the plug is embedded deep in the pore, it may become enlarged and infected, and eventually break through the wall of the pore to inflame the surrounding tissue. The result is an eye-ravaging "swollen cyst" or blemish that causes so many people such—up till now—*cureless* suffering.

Dermatologists now believe that acne is caused by an excess of androgen, a male hormone that to some extent is also present in women. Androgen enlarges the oil glands, spurring them to overproduce. Which is why blemishes are most common during puberty, the time when hormone levels change. Many women have been known to experience flare-ups during their menstrual period, when their hormones are particularly active, and when they begin taking—or stop taking—birth control pills, which contain hormones. Some people break out when they're under stress or when they travel, or when they don't get enough rest, or, according to at least one school of thought, when they eat certain foods. A tendency toward acne is also thought to be hereditary. Whatever—dermatologists now report that more and more adult women are having problems with it.

Recently scientists from the National Cancer Institute discovered that variations of a synthetic derivative of Vitamin A, called synthetic retinoids, in addition to inhibiting the growth of cancer, are able to "drastically reduce the production of sebum in oil glands." Testing thus far has been extremely encouraging—producing very few side effects. It may be a while yet before a cure for acne is developed and marketed—but stay tuned.

## THE ROLE OF DIET

Dermatologists used to single out various foods as causes of acne. They advised patients to stop eating nuts, citrus fruits, shellfish, chocolate, you name it. Recent experiments have proved that diet has little or no effect on acne (with the possible exception of some foods containing iodine). Still, it's a good idea to swear off those foods that you've noticed are directly associated with your breaking out.

Nutritionists, on the other hand, have concluded that a junk-food diet, heavy on sugar and refined foods, will definitely aid and abet bad skin. From experience, I tend to agree. Dermatologists freely (or is that the wrong word to use about these very expensive specialists?) admit that they don't know exactly what causes abnormal hormone activity, or why some people's skins are more sensitive to androgen than other people's. Everybody knows by now that what we eat affects our entire bodies, right down to our glandular and hormonal secretions; in a sense by no means unironic, we *are* what we eat. For example, when we consume too much refined sugar, the pancreas reacts by producing too much of the hormone insulin, and the result can be as drastic as diabetes and hypoglycemia! So when a dermatologist tells you it's okay to eat peanuts and chocolate, that it won't aggravate your acne, you should ask yourself if he's taking into account that you may have been overloading your body with doughnuts, ice cream, white bread, Coca-Cola, and fried chicken since you were *three years old*.

I don't care what the experts say, I still think that if you suffer from bad skin, you owe it to yourself—and to others, who have to look at you—to immediately eliminate as much sugar, refined flour, nuts, fatty meats such as pork and beef, fried foods, and rich dairy products from your diet as you can stand—for at least three months, let's say. If your skin still doesn't improve, at least your figure, digestion, and general health are bound to. But don't be disappointed when you don't wake up the morning after all clear and purified—the toxins from the unhealthy foods you've been eating have been building up in your system for years.

My skin improved dramatically thanks to a model-

211

ing assignment I was on in Portugal with *Bride's* magazine when I was nineteen. The hotel we were staying in didn't have a single dessert on the menu that appealed to me (that's hard to imagine, since by now you know that all desserts appealed to me), and for three weeks I was forced to eat healthy: eggs, fish, vegetables —oh and just a *little* junk food so I wouldn't turn sullen. At the end of the trip, my skin was clearer than it had been since I was a babe. I was beginning to win the battle! Incidentally, on my travels I've noticed that the residents of underdeveloped countries, where refined sugar and flour are not an accepted part of the diet, aren't afflicted with acne; none of the East African tribes I visited had it.

## VISIT A DERMATOLOGIST, PLEASE

Don't try to cure serious skin problems on your own. A change of diet alone won't do it, nor will over-the-counter medications and assorted home remedies. Certain types of skin scar more easily than others, and a serious infection can leave your complexion unevenly pigmented (to put it kindly). So why take the unnecessary risk? A clear skin enhances your appearance far more than an expensive new coat or dress is likely to. Too many people wait far too long before seeking medical help for a disfiguring skin ailment, and just keep hoping against hope that it will vanish all by itself. It won't.

## MAKING DULL SKIN DISAPPEAR

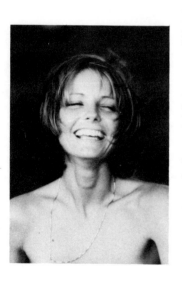

If you don't have the skin you crave, consider this: you may not be taking good enough care of your *body*, because what benefits the body also benefits the skin.

Maybe you're not exercising enough.

The growth of skin cells depends on oxygen and moisture received from the blood. When your circulation is sluggish, your skin receives less nourishment than it needs, and this in turn slows down cell growth and elimination of such waste products as carbon dioxide and fatty acids. So exercise those impurities out of your system; and feel and watch the color and texture of your skin improve along with your blood circulation. A ruddy complexion may be an indication of high blood pressure, and dull or sallow skin of low blood pressure. Exercise can help normalize such irregularities.

Maybe you're not getting enough sleep.

Lack of rest slows down blood circulation to the skin. When I'm tired and tense, my skin looks a sickly gray. Rest refreshes the skin every bit as much as it refreshes the body and mind.

Or maybe you really shouldn't be smoking.

When you smoke, you're doing almost as much harm to your skin as to your lungs—by cutting off the source of oxygen. The nicotine in tobacco causes the small blood vessels in your skin to shrink and thus cuts off circulation. If you continue to smoke, your skin will get duller and coarser as you age. Many experts have hazarded the guess that smoking is partly responsible for crow's-feet around the eyes. That's a heavy trip to lay on smoking, but there you are. Whatever the truth about this calumny proves to be, smoking *can't* be very good for you.

## THE BEST DO-IT-YOURSELF DEEP-CLEANSING FACIAL IN THE WORLD

Aida Thibiant is the most celebrated and sought-after skin-care specialist in all Hollywood. Many a California beauty owes a real debt of thanks to Aida's European techniques and "secret" formulas. I love going to her salon for a deep-cleansing and moisturizing facial. I lie back in a reclining chair, close my eyes (blast and damn the *real* world!), and just totally relax as Aida works on my skin with her practiced hands and sweet-smelling lotions, creams, masques, steam treatments, and unique massages. This is the life they used to lead in palaces—no wonder I feel like a princess. And the results last for weeks.

Ideally, I would like to have a facial by Aida once a month, but I'm usually traveling. I pleaded with her for years to give me her recipe for a special deep cleansing facial that anyone can do for herself, and the other day she divulged it. So here it is, and it's *guaranteed* to give your skin and your psyche a tremendous lift.

Do it before going to bed at night, so your just-cleaned skin can have eight hours to relax, breathe, and otherwise respond to all the good things you've done for it. A do-it-yourself facial takes about an hour, so you'll probably find the time to do it only once a week or so. But that's okay.

There are six basic steps—one or two of them may

turn out to be especially effective, but try to practice them *all* as often as you can.

### 1. The Gommage

*Gommage* is a French word meaning "the erasing of dead cells on the surface of the skin." For this you'll need a cleansing cream that contains lysin, a plant extract that helps melt the dead skin cells, making them easy to remove. Most salon lines of cosmetics carry a cream of this type. Apply it to the skin and wipe it off with cotton balls. If for some unaccountable reason you can't find a gommage cream, begin your facial with step 2.

### 2. Scrubbing and Steaming

Fill a pot with water and add a tablespoon each of the following ingredients: Rosemary (it has great toning properties); camomile (it's relaxing); fennel (it's a decongestant); dried rose buds (they're soothing and sweet-smelling); and camphor (it's both a decongestant and an antibacterial agent). Herbal treatments such as this one are an important part of the European tradition of skin care. Now cover the pot, bring it to a rollicking boil for several minutes, then remove the cover, bend over the pot, and let the sweet-smelling vapor penetrate your pores. Don't cover your head and the pot with a towel—it will only make the concentration of steam too hot, and it *may* irritate your skin and break delicate capillaries. While the steam is cleaning out your pores, massage a honey-almond scrub into your face with gentle, circular movements of your fingertips. (You can make your own scrub by grinding four ounces of blanched almonds in your blender and mixing the powdery meal with four ounces of honey.) Don't pull your skin up and down, and don't massage so roughly that before you know it you've scratched your face. This pure, organic mixture softens up the skin better than any soap I know. And if you haven't eaten in a while, it also *tastes* delicious. Steam and scrub for five minutes, then wipe off the scrub with a washcloth soaked in warm water.

### 3. Toning

Apply a skin freshener to your face with a cotton ball. Aida believes that not even oily-skinned people should use an alcohol-based astringent. "Too harsh for the skin!" is the clarion note of warning she sounds.

### 4. Nourishing

Apply a light-textured cream to your skin with your fingertips. The right cream should not be oily or form a film on top of the skin.

### 5. Pincement Jaquet

This is another French term, meaning "pinching the skin lightly between thumbs and middle fingers." So now, pinch your entire face to step up blood circulation and help the nourishing cream penetrate the skin. Then tap your chin and jaw area with the back of your hand.

### 6. Using a Masque

This is the final step in any facial. Masques shrink your pores, stimulate and nourish your skin, improve your blood circulation, and "trap" the skin's moisture so it can't evaporate. The result is a plumped-up, shining, soft skin that looks young and well rested. The benefits last for several hours after you remove the masque.

#### Quick Money-Saving Masques

1. Beat an egg white with a few drops of lemon juice to tighten your skin.
2. Liquefy a cucumber in the blender with a few drops of lemon juice, which will also help clear your skin.
3. Mix a tablespoon of brewer's yeast with a teaspoon of vegetable oil or water till it's the consistency of a thin gruel (very good for oily skin, but watch out that it doesn't cause dryness and irritation).
4. Soak a couple of cotton pads with the juice of a fresh orange and apply to your skin.

#### Masques for Dry, Delicate Skin

1. Apply plain yogurt to your face.
2. Liquefy an avocado, which is rich in natural oils, in the blender and mix with a few drops of lemon juice.
3. Cooked, cooled oatmeal, which may also be used as a scrub.
4. Liquefy the pulp of a peach in the blender and mix with a few drops of avocado oil or a liquefied mixture of avocado and peach.

Put your masque on, lie back, close your eyes, and enjoy. After fifteen minutes, remove the masque with warm water and a washcloth. Then tone your skin once again with a freshening lotion. Apply a moisturizer or a night cream (and to all a good-night cream!).

## CARING FOR BODY SKIN

The skin on your body, which has far fewer oil glands than the skin on your face, needs special care to stay soft and smooth.

I don't want to cause any anxiety to American mothers, but—here goes: bathing is not always as cleanly and godly as it's been made out to be. In fact, very dry skin improves with less bathing—and in direct proportion to how little you bathe (Pew!).

When I bathe, I try to make the bath a really relaxing experience: I want my nerves calmed as well as my muscles eased and my skin smoothed.

## C.T.'s RECIPE FOR A SENSUOUS BATH

Don't make the water too hot unless your muscles are feeling all achy after an exercise session. Take the phone off the hook, so you won't be tempted to leap out of the tub to answer it. Lower the lights, put on your favorite record, and sip some topsy-turvy champagne.

When I'm in the tub I like to breathe in sweet smells, so I take some of the herbs I used to steam my face, wrap them in a porous cloth bag (a pocket from an old dress or skirt, tied at the top, will do just fine), and float them in the bath. Then I add my favorite fragrant bath oil. It's easy and inexpensive to make your own bath oil—just add a few drops of perfume or oil extract (musk or patchouli oil) to a bottle of unscented coconut or almond oil. This, by the way, was one of Cleopatra's favorite recipes and, as we know, "age cannot wither nor custom stale *her* infinite variety." Stay away from bubble baths that contain drying detergents. Some women like to stir a package of instant powdered milk into the water. To each her own.

Now: Lather your body with a mild soap. The rough surface of a loofa sponge, an aloe fiber bath mit, or a bath brush will slough those dead cells right off your arms and legs.

Wring out a washcloth in the warm water and lay it over your face, gently steaming it. This opens and cleanses the pores, and moisturizes the surface cells as well.

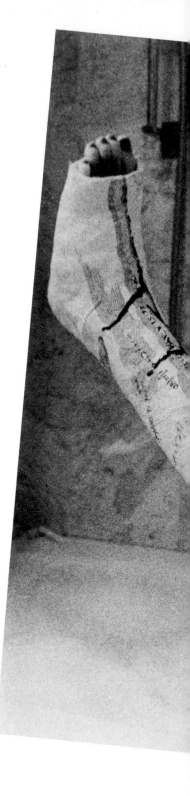

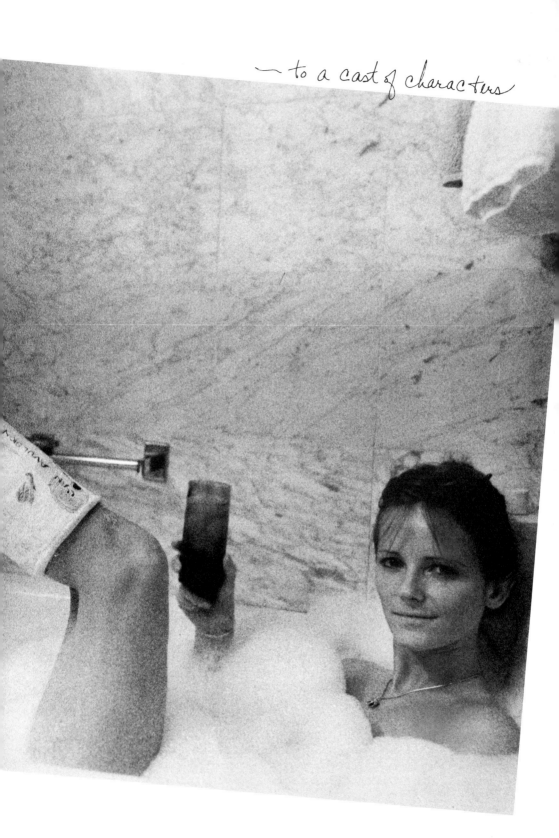

— to a cast of characters

If your legs feel achy, move both hands over the muscles in long, gliding strokes.

But, as one of my favorite Robert Lowell poems puts it: "Dearest, I cannot loiter here in lather like a polar bear." So:

I step out of the tub and immediately I smooth on a generous amount of moisturizer while I'm still damp. The water on my skin helps the moisturizer slide on, especially in the first five minutes after I'm out of the water. Take the extra time to make your bath a real luxury, the snug and watery cradle wherein you gather your thoughts, read a book, write a poem, or hum a favorite tune.

## SKIN TREATMENT PRODUCTS

Because there are rows and rows of skin treatment products on the market, each one of which promises to work miracles, it's awfully hard to distinguish fiction from fact. How, you wonder, will I ever find the one that will work for me? It must exist somewhere, in the heart of that heartless shelf, because you know that others before you have found it.

What I advise is buying a cleanser, toner, and moisturizer all with the same brand name. The cosmetics industry is extremely sophisticated today, and basic products in a single line have been designed by technicians to work together for the good of your skin.

And give the products you select a chance. Unless you're allergic to a lotion or moisturizer, or find it has an instant bad effect on your skin, use it for a month or so before discarding it in favor of another.

Some skin products contain costly ingredients such as fruit extracts, turtle oil, and even mink oil, and there are experts who swear that these additives have no more effect on the skin than do ordinary, down-to-earth cosmetic ingredients such as lanolin and mineral oil. Other experts claim that special oils and extracts can greatly improve your skin. I use a night cream containing an esoteric little substance called collagen, which is a liquid protein that is supposed to firm the skin. There's no denying that expensive products have a scent and texture that are far more enticing than their cheaper counterparts. I mean, who wants to use Crisco on her face?

The most important thing to realize is that no cream yet invented, no matter how expensive it is, can replace a wrinkle with unlined skin. When and how much and how badly you wrinkle is determined largely by hereditary factors and by the amount of time you've spent suicidally overexposing yourself to the sun. Creams soften skin, yes, but they don't perform miracles.

Today, most products are required by law to list on their labels every single ingredient they contain. But unless you happen to know for a fact that you're allergic to some specific substance, the information on the label will be of little use to you because the ingredients usually have indecipherable chemical names— there's no way you're going to know what most of them are or actually do. One thing you can do is avoid alcohol-based products; another is to keep your eye peeled for ingredients like mink that you just know have got to raise the price of the product, or look for those ingredients that you know from past experience will improve your skin.

## HYPOALLERGENIC COSMETICS

A hypoallergenic label doesn't guarantee that the allergy-prone will be immune to every ingredient in the formula. The main difference between hypoallergenic and other products is that the hypos are unscented and packaged under sterile conditions. Many people are allergic to some of the ingredients in perfumes, so using a milder scent will reduce the likelihood of reactions. Here's a Catch-22 for you: you may turn out to be just as allergic to an ingredient in a hypoallergenic product as you are to one in a regular product.

## MAKING YOUR OWN COSMETICS

This is not the greatest idea you never had. It can be very expensive to make your own cosmetics. Besides, homemade products might not work as well, and certainly they won't smell and feel as nice as those you can buy. Given the time it's going to take you to go out and buy the many ingredients necessary for making your own astringent, you'd be better off buying one formulated by professional chemists to last a month or more. But if you're hell-bent on beating the system, then by all means go right ahead and give it a try. But remember, "cosmetics making," like baking and fancy cooking, takes time and energy and doesn't always turn out right.

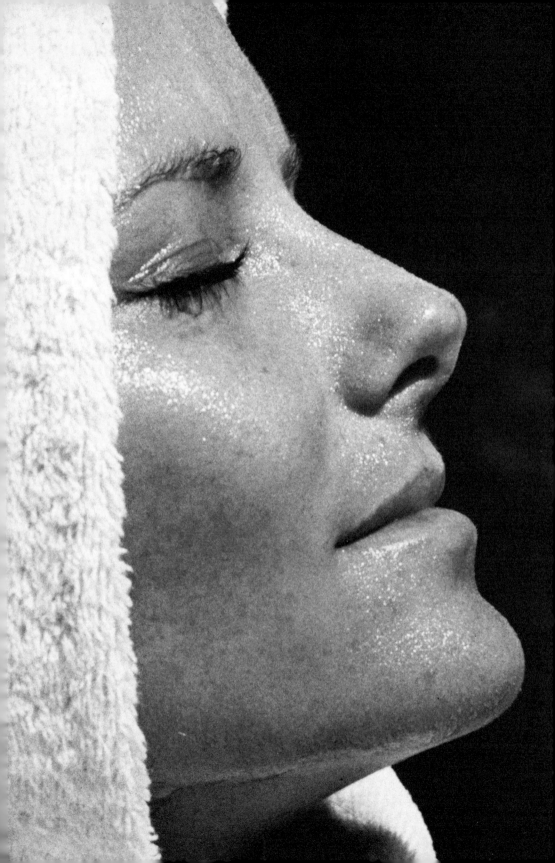

# C.T.'s MINUTE-TO-MINUTE TIPS FOR
## BEAUTIFUL SKIN

### Humidify Your House

A humidifier is one of the best investments you can make if you live in either a very dry climate or a steam-heated house. Hot air absorbs all the moisture it can find, including the moisture in your skin, and can dry out the membrances of your nose and throat. Pans of water near the heating ducts or on the radiators can serve as homemade humidifiers (you can dress them up a bit with rocks or flowers). Or try lowering the thermostat in the winter. And don't forget your plants—they need a squirt of water from time to time, too.

### The Airplane Facial

I am more dependent than most on airplanes, and I'm the first to admit that they have their place in the sun, in the scheme of things, but they certainly were not designed with "saving the skin" in mind. The atmosphere on planes is exceptionally cool and dry, and may dehydrate the skin, mouth, and throat. My little remedy is to drink club soda with lime throughout the trip; and of course I also carry some moisturizer in my purse. I dab a little extra on, even when I'm wearing makeup, so my skin doesn't completely dry out.

### The Breakfast Masque or Guess Who's Coming to Breakfast

If you're alone one morning and want to begin the day with a smooth, glowing skin, then apply a masque at breakfast. There are quick-acting masques on the market which can revitalize your skin in a matter of minutes. Just be sure to wash it off with warm water, and then tone your skin and moisturize.

### Misting Your Face

Living in a humid or foggy climate is great for your complexion (but hell on your clothes and spirit). However, you can create your own moist climate by filling a small spray bottle with mineral water. Or if you're lazy, there are fine mists sold in aerosol cans. Misting will set your makeup and keep your face soft and moist. And also refresh your thoughts, cool you out.

### C.T.'s Telephone Hand Treatment

As the skin on your hands is especially thin and prone to dryness and chapping, you should apply hand lotion

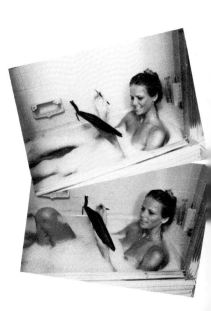

throughout the day. The way I remember to do this is by keeping a small bottle by the telephone. Every time I see that little bottle staring at me, reproaching me for my dereliction, I rub some lotion in.

### C.T.'s Luscious Lips Insurance Policy

Don't let sleeping lips lie—they're sensitive, and they need your protection in order to stay soft and moist. I use a lip protection stick all year 'round under lipstick or gloss. Another way to moisturize lips is to wet them with a damp washcloth and then apply a gloss. Lips burn in the sun, so if you spend a lot of time out-of-doors, use a lip protector or look for a lipstick that contains a sun block.

### The Water Cure

My skin tends to dry out when I'm tense and reeling from the pace of life in New York ("There's a neurosis in the air that the inhabitants mistake for energy," is how Evelyn Waugh described New York's vibes in his novel *Brideshead Revisited*), or when I've spent too much time in wildly overheated rooms. What I do then is go to the water faucet every chance I get, and drink down as much water as I can. After just a few days of this internal moisturizing treatment, my skin is smooth again.

## MISTAKES PEOPLE MAKE

### Sun Baking

These days, there is nothing more OUT than a dark, leathery tan. Baking your body in the sun without using a sun-blocking lotion is the best recipe for both wrinkling your skin and contracting skin cancer. The consensus among dermatologists is that the *only* effective method for keeping skin smooth and young is to protect it from the sun as much as humanly possible. I'm an active person with a genuine love of the out-of-doors and I refuse point blank to swathe myself in scarves and hats. But I wouldn't dream of not applying a good sunscreen with PABA to the exposed parts of my body, along with nosecoat, before facing the sun. The sun-block deflects the sun's damaging rays and at the same time allows me to get a light tan that actually protects my skin. If you do get sunburned, here's what to do: draw a tepid bath, and add two cups of oatmeal

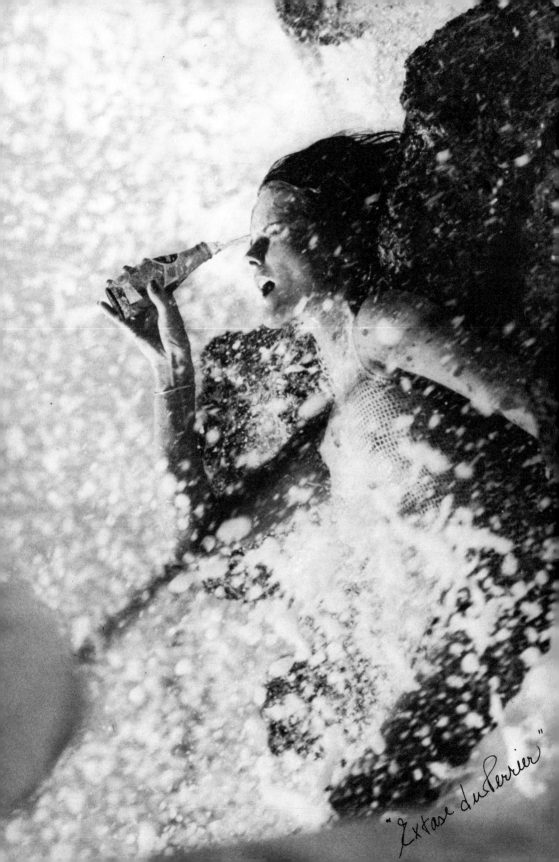

"Extase du Perrier"

to the water—and, as they say in the comic strips, *no soap*. Afterwards, apply a heavy cream to your wet skin, followed by a masque consisting of one ounce yogurt and one ounce buttermilk. It's as soothing as it sounds.

## Sun Protection

Baby oil does a good job pampering and lubricating your skin but when it comes to protecting you from the sun, forget it. Ditto for mineral oil, and even for some of the highly touted suntanning oils on the market. To guard against sun damage, you'll have to buy a sun block containing PABA. The only natural oil capable of adequately protecting your skin from the sun is sesame oil.

## Too Much of a Good Thing

Women who apply countless creams and medications to their skin—who steam it, masque it, and buff it as if it were a pair of penny loafers—run the risk of ending up with drier, duller, or oilier skins than women who practice the little praised art of sensible moderation. Too much steaming and hot-water cleansing can stimulate your oil glands to overproduce, which in turn can aggravate an acne condition; too much buffing can remove the cells that serve to protect the skin; and too much moisturizing can clog your pores and give your skin an altogether dull finish. Yes of course, work for a beautiful skin, just so long as you don't make the common mistake of thinking that more means better.

## Overfocusing on a Blemish

When I was having problems with, ahem, "grog-blossoms," I used to think about them all the time, and even a single "blossom" could make me feel terribly self-conscious; my whole world was circumscribed by that "flaw." Now, when the inevitable happens from time to time, I try to remember that it's my entire face that people will see, not just the "spot." So if your skin breaks out, remember this: others will be focusing on your eyes or your smile or your facial expressions and probably won't even notice the "trouble."

## When to Have a Professional Facial

A facial does not always improve your skin right away; sometimes, when the treatment of blemishes is involved, the skin becomes temporarily redder and more inflamed. So schedule your facial for at least a day or two before a special occasion.

### Using Tissues on Your Face

Don't ever use tissues to apply creams, lotions, or toners; they contain tiny woody fibers that will scratch your skin. Use cotton balls or pads.

### The Danger of Believing Everything You Read

There is enough propaganda about skin products and skin care around today to overwhelm, if not actually bury, you. It seems as if every dermatologist and cosmetician in the world is flogging a different system of skin care— each of them completely foolproof. It's no wonder that so many people are confused. All you have to remember is that the best judge of what's good for your skin is, first and finally, you.

So: experiment (within limits), and *observe* how your skin is responding. Before long, you too will be comfortable and safe in your own saved skin.

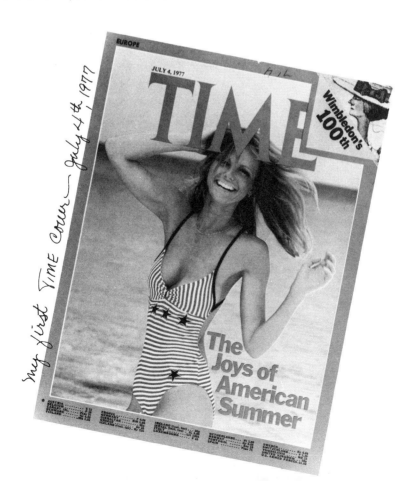

my first Time cover— July 4th, 1977

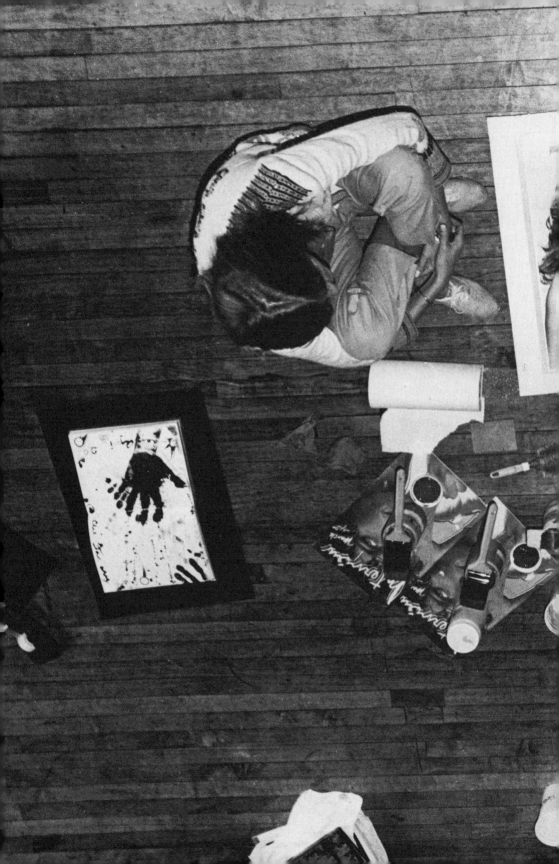

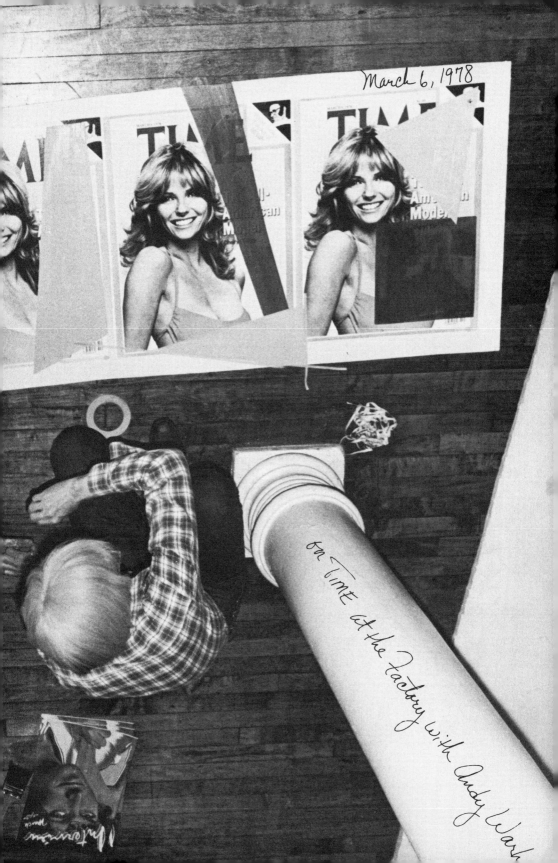

March 6, 1978

on Time at the Factory with Andy Warhol

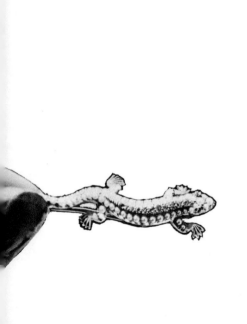

# 8

# Life Is, a Dressy Occasion: How to Get It Right

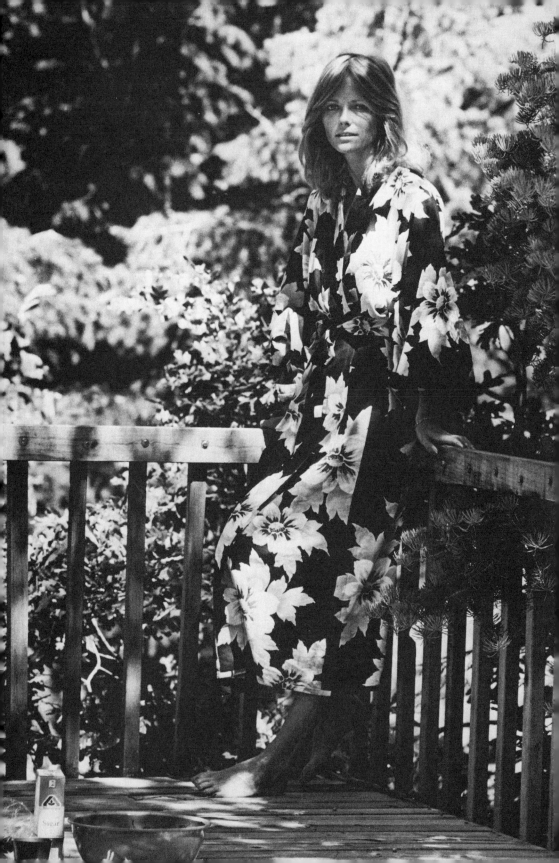

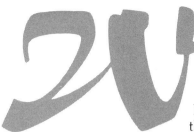

e all know women who go to great expense and trouble to dress very badly and, what's more, "derive a kind of puzzling authority from it." The woman who knows her stuff takes care to choose clothes that communicate her unique self to the people she encounters; she knows that, as Virginia Tiger has written, "clothes may make the man but woman *is* the world she wears." She uses her clothes to enhance her best features and draw attention away from, if not artfully conceal, her second-best. She realizes that fashion is not only a mysterious but a very revealing form of human expression. If she *really* wants to dress to kill she'll wear clothes that run toward greater and greater simplicity so that people notice *her* rather than *them*.

Most women have a closetful of clothes, and yet they're never satisfied with what they have; they spend a lot of unnecessary time and money shopping for the latest styles—often not even bothering to insure that the clothes go well together. Others summarily (and boldly, given that life itself is a dressy occasion) dismiss fashion altogether, in favor of comfortable old standbys—till the day when a job interview or something equally momentous pounces and they panic because they have—and how many times have you heard or said these words yourself?—"nothing to wear." (And, if she's the world she wears, just what does *that* make her? No, fashion is not at all as frivolous as it looks.)

■ *Do you find yourself buying new clothes and then almost never wearing them?*

■ *Do you buy new clothes only to discover that you have nothing in your wardrobe to complement them?*

■ *Do you shop only before special occasions—and then frantically, like one possessed?*

■ *Do you feel your clothes are out of style, uninteresting, or inappropriate?*

■ *Do you shop only in the budget departments of local stores because you've convinced yourself that you can't afford designer clothes?*

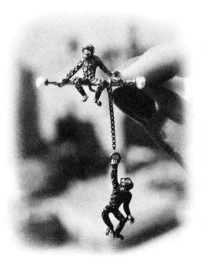

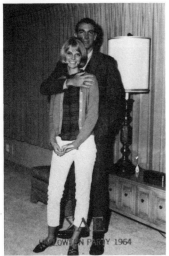

1964

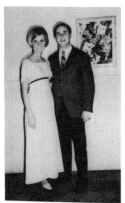

1965

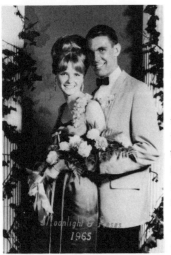

1965

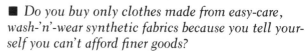

■ *Do you buy only clothes made from easy-care, wash-'n'-wear synthetic fabrics because you tell your-self you can't afford finer goods?*

If you've answered yes to any of the above questions, it will pay you many times over to read the rest of this chapter.

First of all, I've always felt that so-called good taste is something that anyone with a head on her shoulders can learn. Subscribing to a fashion magazine is one way to begin—notice I said "begin," because you don't want to let the fashion magazines have complete dominion over what you wear. I look to them for guidance and new ideas.

One of the biggest discoveries I made was that updating a wardrobe is not as expensive or time-consuming as is commonly thought. Even if you really can't afford designer dresses, you should try them on anyway, if only to see firsthand what a beautiful cut and a tasteful fabric can do for you. It's not a wasted day when you discover, as I did quite late in the game, that clothes made from beautiful fabrics are not as far out of your price range as you imagined and that they're just as economical to care for as those grungy synthetic wash-'n'-wear materials.

In fashion, it's the overall effect that counts. The truly well-dressed woman will look just as smart in casual wear as she will in formal evening clothes. She has learned, probably by trial and error (few of us have unerring instincts), which color combinations, textures, and fabrics are the most flattering to her skin and hair and personality.

## THE WAY I DRESSED BACK THEN

Every time someone compliments me on my "fashion sense," I have to stop and sort of pinch myself, because until very recently it never even occurred to me that I had any. I went through most of my life not knowing what to wear, or even what I really wanted to wear. As far as clothes went, I more or less ran with the pack. A few years ago, however, I began to wake up to the fact that fashion sense is not a special talent some women are born with and others are not, but rather—like most other things—a matter of effort, self-education, and—again, trial and error.

All through my teens I stuck to the most conservative styles and rarely strayed from the color blue (actually, truth to tell, it's still my favorite color). When I began to model and came into contact with the fashion world, I developed enough self-assurance to experiment a little with clothes. I said a faint good-bye to the safe approach—a little too quickly, as it turned out, because—I can tell you—I had my fair share of disasters. I'll never forget the time I went out and spent a fortune on a pair of special plastic see-through, high-heeled shoes. Oh they were the last word—or the next-to-last, anyway—and I felt proud of being brave enough to sport a pair. I put them right on and went to a fraternity party. After I was on my dancing, sweating tootsies for only about an hour, those chic plastic attention-getters steamed up and clouded over so you couldn't tell my toes from twigs. My ungracious chums slapped their knees over the hilarity of it all—making me even more self-conscious (if that were possible). One of them even had the nerve to ask me if the shoes had come complete with windshield wipers! I *almost* managed to be formidable in my distress.

Another time, I really branched out and got a wonderful pink mini-dress, which I wore with white knee socks, flat shoes, and a little pink purse. All dolled up (literally!), I was sure I looked more "in style" than anyone on campus. As I strolled along to English class, my cute little purse got caught in my cute white knee socks and it took me half an hour to disentangle the various parts of my oh-so-fashionable outfit— much to the amusement of passing students.

When I began to model for *Glamour*, I found my mentor in fashion editor Julie Britt. She had a great flair for clothes, and soon I was slavishly copying everything she wore. If Julie came to a shooting in a beautifully fitted A-line dress and Gucci shoes, I'd rush out and buy an A-line dress and buckled shoes that looked as much like Gucci as I could afford. I wouldn't buy anything without first asking myself "Would Julie buy this?" or "Would Julie ever wear that?" There's no question I learned a lot from Julie, but copying is never as edifying as developing a sense of style of your own.

For years I would wear anything I could see was in fashion regardless of how it looked on *me*. I kept telling myself: "I must above all things be snazzy." So I wore the hip-hugger pants and the skintight tops that were so popular in the sixties (despite the fact that I was then pretty heavy, and long-waisted to boot). I also followed the crowd and wore the most extreme versions of the mini-skirt, although at the time my legs were far too thick to be out there where everyone could see them.

As a model I was constantly being exposed to the most beautiful clothes created by the top designers. It was like pressing your nose up against the window of your very favorite pastry shop—temptation incarnate. When I was a very naïve twenty-one, I bought an incredibly snazzy, very expensive, vampy black dress—slit all the way up. In the designer's showroom the dress had made me look like the glamorous, soignée woman I thought I wanted to be. I coveted it, so I bought it. But when I got it home and tried it on in front of my tell-me-no-lies mirror, I saw that it made me look like a little girl wearing a costume. It was a gorgeous, languorous dress, but better leave it alone, Cheryl, I said to myself, it isn't for you. I had a hard enough time getting up the nerve to take it back.

## THE WAY I DRESS NOW

Now that at least to a certain extent I've developed a fashion sense of my own, I realize that I feel most comfortable in classic and simple clothes for daytime wear. Who wants to get all dressed up in the morning, anyway?

I prefer to put on one outfit that I know will get me through the whole day. Well-cut jeans in different fabrics, one-of-a-kind silk shirts, T-shirts, classically tailored skirts and blazers, vests and sweaters in subtle colors—these are my favorites for daytime. I'm a strong believer in wearing parts of the same outfit several days running (but not, however, if you've been running for several days!)—a common practice in Europe, by the way—but with different accessories; that way, I don't have to make a decision about what goes with what *every* morning. I prefer the milder styles to offbeat, zany outfits, because coming up with a really successful offbeat look takes a lot of time, thought, "creativity," and also, unless you get it exactly right, it usually comes out exactly wrong. Whatever fashion imagination I do have blossoms at night (in this sense, I'm quite the opposite of a morning glory), when I can spare the time to put some real effort and ingenuity into the way I dress. I love the fantasy aura of evening clothes—shiny fabrics, satins, velvets, rhinestone belts, and high, strappy, sexy sandals. One of my favorite outfits for a champagne evening (which you can have either with or without the champagne) is a pair of tight turquoise velvet jeans that I wear with my shameless purple fox fur. There's also a shimmery sequined traffic-stopping silk shirt that I love—it's a hot

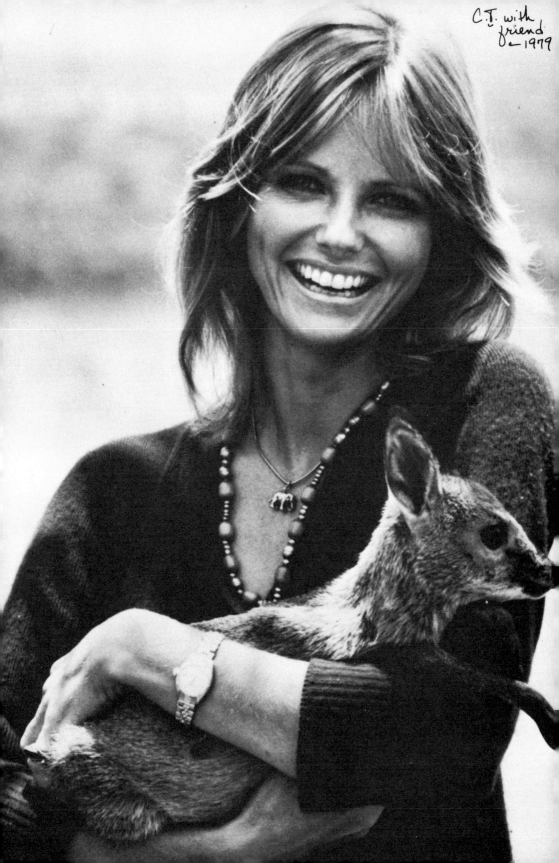

C.J. with friend — 1979

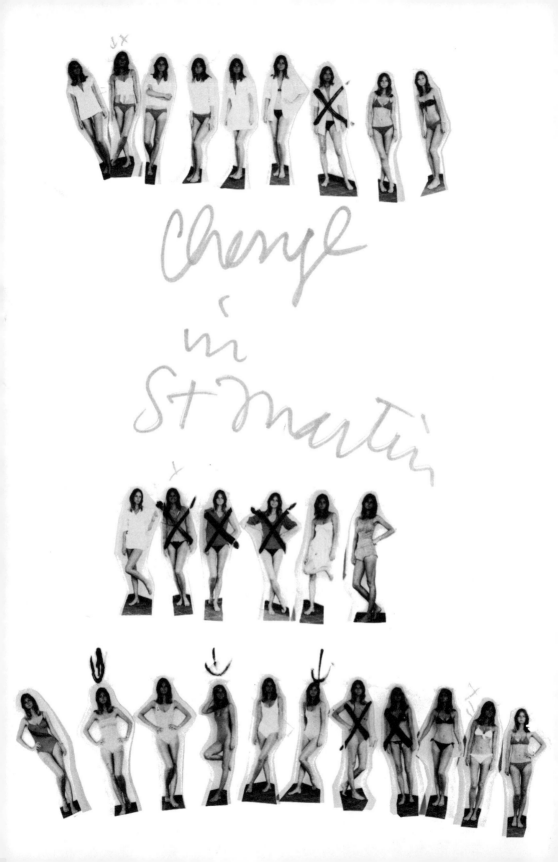

shade of rose and I wear it with white satin pants and gold sandals: ooh-la-la.

Because I'm sometimes in the eye of the public, I *have* to own more clothes than the average person; but I still don't believe in overdoing it, and my wardrobe happens to be smaller than that of most of my friends. I have a great weakness for anything from that classic American designer Calvin Klein, and from St. Laurent, whose imaginative designs have refurbished the fantasy lives of so many women the world over ("grasshopper notes of genius!"). I adore Ann Klein's colors and fabrics and Oscar de la Renta's fabulous evening silks, and Giorgio Armani's elegant *and* practical clothes. Another of my big fashion heroes is the inimitable Halston. These designers are all friends of mine and they have all helped teach me to select and appreciate what looks good on me.

Here are some suggestions for how to develop *a new approach to what you wear* (kind of a long-winded way of saying "fashion sense").

## FIND A MENTOR

As I've said, my fashion mentor was Julie Britt, and you should be so lucky. If you know a beautifully dressed woman, someone whose fashion sense you admire, watch what she wears, notice how she combines colors and fabrics, how she puts her clothes together, and how she uses jewelry, belts, and scarves. Observe how she chooses clothing to display her figure and coloring to their best advantage. Don't only ask her advice, try to get her to come along with you on your next shopping trip. I bet she developed her fashion sense through careful thought and study, and not through any accident. Even now, I "study" the women I consider exceptionally well-dressed. I no longer feel the need to copy what they're wearing but I'm still very much open to ideas and inspiration; I may go out and buy a particular dress I've seen them wear—but only if I think it will look right on me, and then what I'll do is wear it with completely different accessories and in a different way from them, because no two women wear a dress the same way. Your goal, then, should be not to copy but to discover what exactly it is that governs how well-dressed women dress.

## SUBSCRIBE TO FASHION MAGAZINES

As I travel throughout the country, I'm surprised to see how few women are aware of what the current style is. And there's really no excuse for this; the many excellent fashion magazines published here and abroad can keep every woman up to date. Their function is to educate you to absorb from them and to help you catalyze (not cauterize) your own ideas.

I used to get awfully discouraged leafing through the fashion magazines, looking at models like Verushka in her height and glory. I would think, "Are you kidding? I could never look like that in a million years." Now, of course, I realize that I'm not supposed to look like the layout in a fashion magazine (unless of course it's me, Cheryl Tiegs, who's in it). Don't attempt to reproduce the outfits you see, don't strive and toil to look like the model on the page. Believe me, she's *too* put together for everyday life, she's a living doll, just perfect—for a dollhouse! Fashion layouts are designed to provide a fantasy-inducing ambience, and the *last* thing they should be taken for is a prescription for reality. So use them wisely. Let them suggest new lines and styles to you—broader shoulders, narrower pants, an authentic peasant image, or the sleek, glamorous look, whatever. They're meant to give you ideas that you then modify to suit yourself. Let's say the look for spring is the va-va-voom "gypsy look" complete with shawls, petticoats, turbans, full skirts, ruffles, and bangles. This may give you the license you need to bring a shawl with you in the evening, or get your old full skirt out of the back closet. Pay attention to the silhouettes, fabrics, and colors the magazines are promoting, then decide which of the current trends are right for *your* figure and *your* personality. It's a mistake to totally ignore current trends; being rabidly anti-fashion may be chic—for about ten minutes!

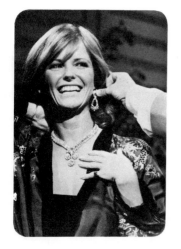

## SHOP WITHOUT BUYING

If you're dissatisfied with your wardrobe, yet can't imagine an alternative, experiment in your local department store and boutiques. Try on styles and fabrics you've never worn before. Put together unusual combinations. Try on designer clothes you know you could never afford, and evening clothes you think you'd never wear. Have a ball. Indulge yourself. Be bold—but not too bold: leave your checkbook and credit cards at home or in your back pocket. Your mission this trip is not mission impossible, because you're there not to buy but to discover. Keep your eyes on the mirror, that's you in there—look at yourself realistically. Your goal is to see what *different* clothes can do for you, so don't stick obstinately to old favorites, don't be a donkey—new vistas are opening up before you. By examining what is available, without feeling the psychological pressure to buy, you'll form a new impression of yourself in relation to fashion with a capital "F." Later, think over the different yous that you saw in the mirror and ask yourself how you felt about each of them. Then—and only then—return to the shop and make your selections.

## WHICH COMPLIMENTS TO TAKE AT FACE VALUE

When you have something new on, listen carefully—and discriminatingly—to what others have to say about it. Don't fish for compliments—the heartfelt ones will come of their own accord and you'll know them when you hear them. Sometimes the admiring (or envious) expression in a friend's eyes will tell you more than an over-enthusiastic exclamation.

## ANALYZING YOUR CLOTHES

Make it a point to analyze the clothes you have before going out and buying new ones. Many people fail to make good enough use of the clothes they already own. These are the same people who make the same mistakes every time they shop.

### List Your All-Time Favorites

Everybody has her favorite outfit that she wears and wears and wears because she knows she always looks good in it. One of my favorites was a black silk St. Laurent shirt, which I'd purchased in the men's shop. I wore it till the cuffs were practically in shreds and the collar was completely, triumphantly frayed. Think about clothes you've owned that you loved and wore into extinction. Which clothes in your closet right this minute get the most wear? Why? You'll probably find that your favorites all have a similar mood, style, or fabric. Ask yourself why you love these particular clothes, and how you felt about them when you bought them. Sometimes it's the dress you were ambivalent about in the store that spends the least time in your closet. It may be that the clothes you love are connected to happy moments.

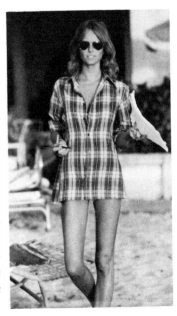

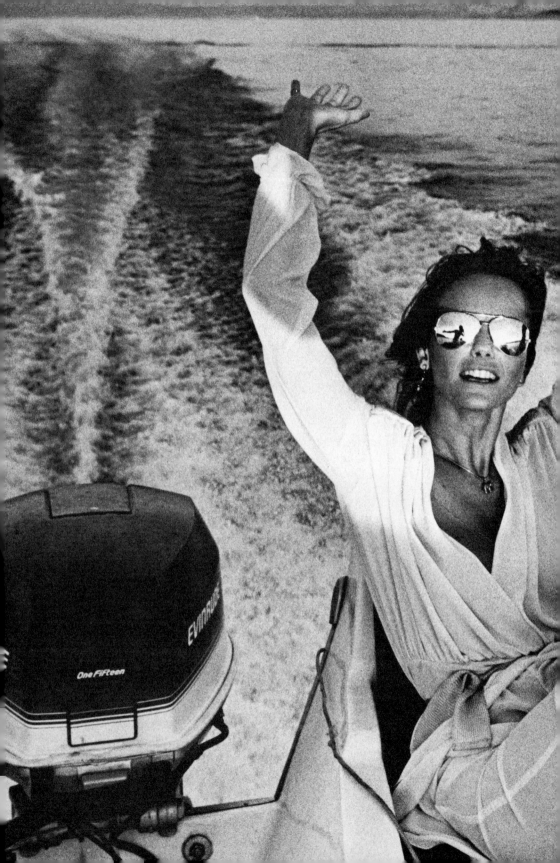

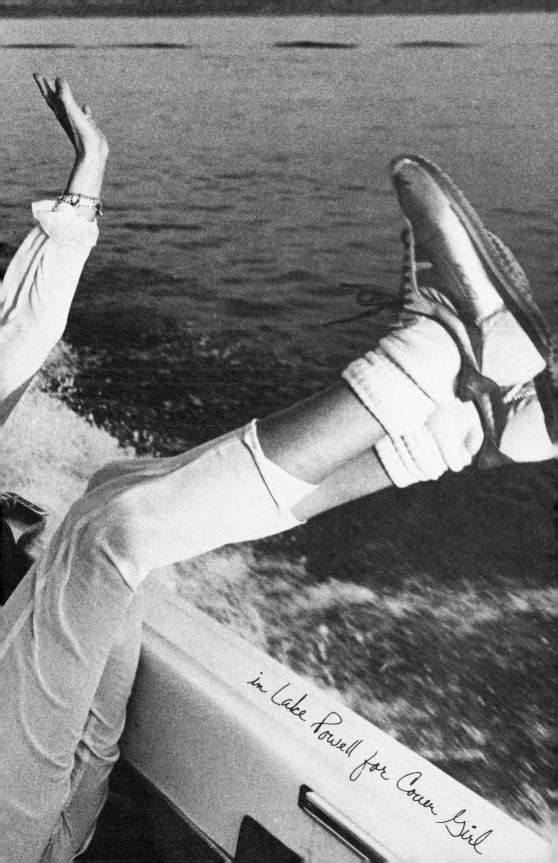

in Lake Powell for Cover Girl

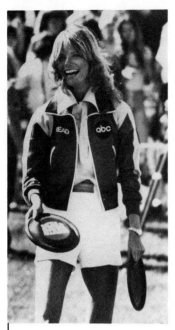

## LIST YOUR MISTAKES (ONE TO TEN THOUSAND)

Go ahead, don't hang back—make a list of the clothes you bought that wound up hanging unworn in the back of your closet. Take the extravagant white Austrian peasant dress with the lace-up bodice that I bought five or six years ago. It looked wonderful, positively irresistible, in the designer's showroom. I wore it once and felt like a misplaced milkmaid. When you're in a store, surrounded on all sides by exciting fashions, your fancies and fantasies can often get the better of you and you may buy something that really has no place in your life (as you discover sooner rather than later). Or your mistakes may take the form of choosing colors that once they are on you, you find too flamboyant for comfort, or very tailored clothes that seemed perfect for the job but make you feel unfeminine after working hours. And clothes whose textures irritate your skin, or those that don't fit well, no matter how beautiful they are, are always a mistake. Analyzing the kind of mistake you're likely to make will make you less prone to making those mistakes again.

### Giving Away the Clothes You Never Wear

A lot of women keep their closets full to bursting with clothes they would never in this life be caught dead in. The mistakes hanging there may be expensive ones, but give them away. Be generous. It may help to remember that clothes that have gone out of style seldom come back in; if you're sick of something, don't keep it in the bound-to-be-blasted hope that you'll see it resurrected five years hence in the pages of *Bazaar*.

## BUYING NEW CLOTHES

Shopping is a bore—and can be a trauma—for many women; for others it's an obsession, a compulsion second to none, an actual demon. Some women buy clothes they can't really wear because they have a warped self-image—they see themselves as younger, older, fatter, thinner, or more or less sophisticated than they really are. Some get high on the atmosphere in the store and buy clothes that will never fit properly. Millions and millions of dollars—*your* dollars—go down the drain every year, courtesy of all the clothes you soon decide you don't want, need, or enjoy.

Department stores have always kind of overwhelmed me. I feel the same way when I'm in a fancy restaurant and a waiter hands me a menu so big it blocks out the whole world. Working for ABC, I couldn't afford to remain oblivious to fashion—I mean, it's part of my job to be in style—so every year, in the spring and in the fall, I update my limited wardrobe. In Los Angeles I gravitate to two boutiques, Maxfield Blue and Charles Galley, where I know the sales personnel and they know me, which I like. I will occasionally go out of my way to shop for an evening dress, something with a melting effect. Over the years I've picked up or invented some shopping tricks and techniques that may be of some help to you as you go about the potentially killing business of building a wardrobe within your price range.

## UPDATING YOUR WARDROBE

It is definitely not necessary—or "NN," as a good friend of mine always says—to buy a whole new wardrobe every year in order to stay in the so-called swim. You should be able to successfully combine a few new things with the clothes you already own. But before shopping, go through your closet and single out the outfits you're really going to wear that year. Make a list of styles, colors, and accessories that would go well with the clothes you have. When you hit your favorite boutique or department store, look for the type of clothes in the colors and fabrics you've determined you need. And whatever you do, don't buy something just because it's marked down.

When I buy clothes, I always lay them out on the counter and mentally combine them with the clothes I have at home, before I even take them into the fitting room.

## FABRICS

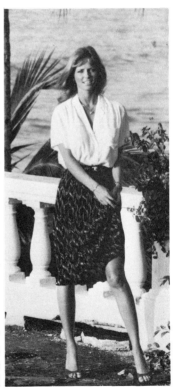

Fabrics should never be underestimated. Everybody loves the feel of soft clothes and few can stand fabrics that are rough or itchy to the touch. A beautiful fabric makes the person who's wearing it feel sensuous, and has even been known to make other people want to reach out and touch it. I go so far as to automatically write off clothes that even *look* as if they might be irritating; a scratchy-looking unlined jacket or a coarse sweater communicates a downright uncomfortable feeling—anyway, that's the message *I* get. Another plus for soft, flowing fabrics is that they reveal the lines of your body as you move in a way that's—frankly—sexy. Whenever I buy a dress or skirt, I choose a fabric that subtly reveals the shape of my legs.

## How to Judge

You have to educate your fingertips to tell the difference between a fine fabric and an inferior one. A good material should feel soft, cool, luxurious. The better it feels, the better it most probably is. Cottons, silks, wools, linens, and synthetics are all made in different weaves and grades. Silk is a strong, long-lasting fiber, whatever grade it is, but the finest weaves will feel as soft as butter. A good wool garment will also feel good enough to eat, and it has the added advantage of not wrinkling easily. Anything made of fine wool will hang in a neat line and fold smoothly. Material that's 100 percent cotton is finer in texture and wears better than a combination of cotton and synthetic blends. I prefer natural fabrics, but there are some modern synthetic materials that are very fine and resemble silks or elegant cottons. Rayons, for example, are made from tree fibers and are nice and soft, and rayon and acetate blends combine into a beautiful fabric that also feels good. Some polyesters, a material often used by designers, feel and look exactly like silk, satin, or polished cotton. Here again, use C.T.'s twenty-second touch test to identify a fine synthetic; the best of them will feel luxurious and slither between your fingertips, while a poor-quality one will be practically untouchable.

Good fabrics, needless to say, are more expensive and require a bit more care than poor-quality ones—as they should. In my opinion, this country places far too much emphasis on practicality—with the result that both men and women in droves buy polyester drip-dry-type synthetics that feel and look cheap and stiff. I strongly encourage you to purchase the best fabric, even if it means you have to settle for fewer things. You will look sexier and more elegant in beautiful fabrics, and they'll certainly last longer.

"What about my dry-cleaning bills?" you're probably

getting ready to ask. Contrary to popular belief, good fabrics don't really have to be dry-cleaned, even when they're labeled "Dry clean only." Silks and fine fabrics were invented eons before the dry-cleaning industry was even a gleam in somebody's avaricious eye, and they can perfectly well be washed by hand. Most silk blouses, fine synthetics, linens, rayons, wool sweaters, and even cashmeres can be laundered in *cold* water and Woolite. And there's a good all-fabric bleach for hard-to-remove stains. Washing, in fact, gets fabrics cleaner than dry-cleaning, which in the long run can be destructive to fine silks.

## HOW CLOTHES ARE CUT

A good garment is both well-cut and well-made. Here are a few techniques of workmanship to be on the lookout for.

A *properly set zipper* should lie flat and even. If the zipper is puckered or curling, chances are the entire garment has been sloppily put together and won't ever hang right.

A *well-sewn seam* sometimes has two lines of stitching. If the item you're planning to buy is torn along the seam, turn your back on it, even if it looks like it can be easily mended—it has either not been well made or not been inspected.

*Hems* of a skirt or dress should hang evenly (many don't), and the stitching should be secure.

*Consider the fit.* Too many women buy clothes for style or color without bothering to take into consideration the way they're cut or how they fit. Unless something fits, and fits well, it won't do much for you no matter which fashion luminary designed it or how much it cost. If you would like to be a smaller size, *diet*; then buy clothes that fit you. Don't, as some diet experts recommend, buy a smaller size dress than you take—as an "inspiration" or incentive—it may never quite fit your reduced contours and you'll have thrown your money away.

*Pants.* Let's face it—I have—most of us have trouble finding pants that fit. Fortunately, pants can usually be altered by the tailor at your local dry cleaner's for a reasonable fee. Make sure they fit properly in the hips and crotch; bend and sit in them to see if they're comfortable. If the hips fit, but the waist or crotch is too loose, a tailor can easily take the pants in along the back seam and in the legs. Never buy pants (or any

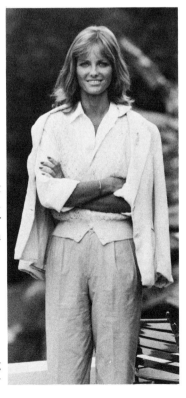

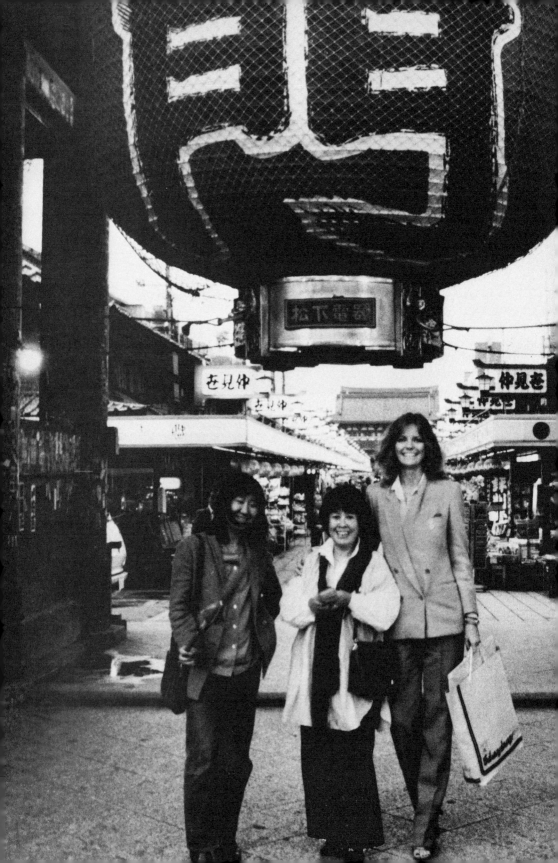

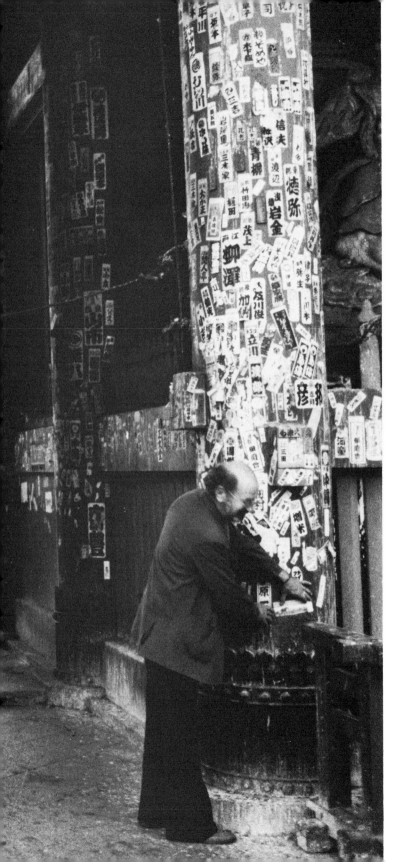

247

Shopping in
Tokyo 1979

garment, for that matter) that are too tight, planning to "let them out." Clothes are not as amply made today as they used to be, and it is all but impossible to make them larger. As for length, pants just have to be the right length or forget it. When you shop for them, wear the type of heel you want to wear with them. Shoes with different heels can't as a rule be worn with the same pants. This is a small point, I grant you, but oh what a difference it can make.

*Shirts, Jackets, and Sweaters.* I like the look of a blouse, sweater, or jacket that's reasonably tight under the arm—it gives a neater, rangier, girl-of-the-limber-lost look, with the seam of the shoulder falling on top of the shoulder line. When you're buying a jacket, make sure the hem falls beneath the buttocks, because if it's any shorter, it will tend to look too small. The cuffs of a jacket should be short enough for the blouse underneath to show. As James Cagney once said, "I like to show a lot of linen." (This was maybe after he shoved that grapefruit in Mae Clark's face.) If you have on a short-sleeved blouse, just push the jacket sleeves up above the elbows.

*The Cut of the Garment on the Figure You Cut or Cut Up in.* A well-designed, well-cut dress—and the two are for all practical purposes synonymous—should be able to be worn in a certain size by many differently shaped bodies. As I've said before—and brace yourself, I'm going to say it again, the only way to learn what well-cut clothes can do for you is to try them on; from time to time, it will pay off to pay more and go for quality instead of quantity.

What I admired most about Julie Britt's wardrobe was its dramatic simplicity. I made a point of learning how she achieved the effect she did. One time, during a *Glamour* trip to Paris, she took me shopping and taught me, as only she could, to appreciate the difference between a Sonia Rykiel sweater and an ordinary one. And, let's not kid ourselves, there *is* a difference. Designer names and prices may not be in our league but that's no reason to automatically reach for the copies. This is going to sound as old as the rushes of the Nile: *use your own creativity* (ten to one you've got some if you only knew it) and be your *own* original.

## YOUR, AHEM, BUDGET

Judiciousness—that's the key requirement here. You don't have to be rich to be well-dressed—remember what I said before about women who go to great expense and trouble and come out dressed "importantly" but very badly. Not that good clothing is cheap—those who want a beautiful wardrobe have to be prepared to invest their fashion dollar carefully. My best cut and most expensive clothes are the ones I can wear year in and year out without wearing *them* out because they're so well made. I advise buying fewer garments but ones of good design instead of accumulating a large trendy wardrobe that is doomed to eventual, if not instant, obsolescence. Some traditional clothes, like your good old Chanel, stay in fashion forever, for what is a tradition, anyway, but a fashion that has lasted? On the other hand, the silhouette of skirts, dresses, and pants may change in the course of a single season. Obviously it is more practical to spend money on garments that will stay in style at least long enough to stabilize your wardrobe (these shaky days a wardrobe is one of the few things you *can* stabilize—barring earthquakes, tidal waves, and other natural phenomena).

## HOW TO KNOW WHAT TO BUY

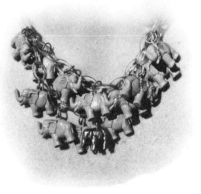

Me, I always know when I want to buy something. I remember reading in high school that the critic and anthologist William Rose Benét knew when a poem was good when the hairs on the back of his neck began bristling. And it's something like that with me and clothes. By now I have sort of a bristle-sense for the kinds of clothes that suit me best. If you have to keep asking yourself, "Do I need it? Do I even really want it? Does it *really* look good on me?" you probably shouldn't get it. It helps to get to know salespeople in the stores you frequent. The people who work in the shops I go to the most often know my tastes at least as well as I do. I've gotten to the point where I can rely on them and just disappear into a dressing room and wait for them to present me with the latest goodies, and they have yet to disappoint or betray me. If you're trying to change your "fashion image" and can't decide whether or not something looks good on you, take along a friend whose taste you trust. Apart from whatever advice she gives you, she'll make the whole business more like a junket.

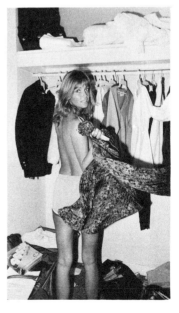

## HOW TO CREATE AN "ORIGINAL" OUTFIT

Even if you do have a closetful of pretty clothes, maybe you don't have the know-how to put them together in terrific combinations. Here are some suggestions that might just work.

## Select the Silhouettes That Flatter Your Proportions

Since few people's figures are ideally proportioned, to look good in clothes they are going to have to wear styles and combinations that emphasize the best parts of their figures and give the desired illusion—whether of thinness, fullness, or longer lines. Here's a rough guide to putting together outfits geared to your particular figure.

*Heavy:* If you're heavy or big-boned, avoid both skintight clothes and voluminous, tent-like garments because neither is going to make you look smaller. Fairly loose clothes, with tops that fall from the shoulder, will give the illusion of softness and length. And so will V-necks. Lines should be relaxed and flowing, fabrics should be fluid. For the full figure, well-tailored clothes are a must. Pants should have a smooth front and a natural waistline. Don't make the mistake I did of buying pleated pants—they only added fullness at a time when my old thin self was in exile. Avoid pants with a high waistband, baggy pants, and again and above all, tight pants. And, if you don't like the size of your backside, don't buy pants with large back pockets.

*Thin:* The Duchess of Windsor is reputed to have said, "You can never be too rich or too thin." Well, she was wrong—about the thin part. You *can* be too thin, at least for some styles of clothes. If certain parts of your body—chest, collarbones, legs—are spare and bony, what are you waiting for? For Heaven's sake, cover them up! And stay away from halters, low necks, bare midriffs, and short shorts. Go for full-cut clothing in textured fabrics to fill out the curves of your body. If you're partial to straight skirts or skintight jeans, then wear a top with soft, full lines. You should be able to wear pants that are exaggeratedly full at the waistline. Almost all clothes look better when draped on a thin figure.

*Short:* If you're small, short jackets, narrow skirts, and pants with straight-cut legs and high waistbands are a safe bet to make your legs look longer. Also wear your skirts a few inches below the knee if you want to make your legs look longer. Such accessories as heavy jewelry, big purses, broad-brimmed hats, and bulky mufflers will bury you. Also avoid T-strap, thick ankle strap, or chunky-heeled shoes, because they'll give

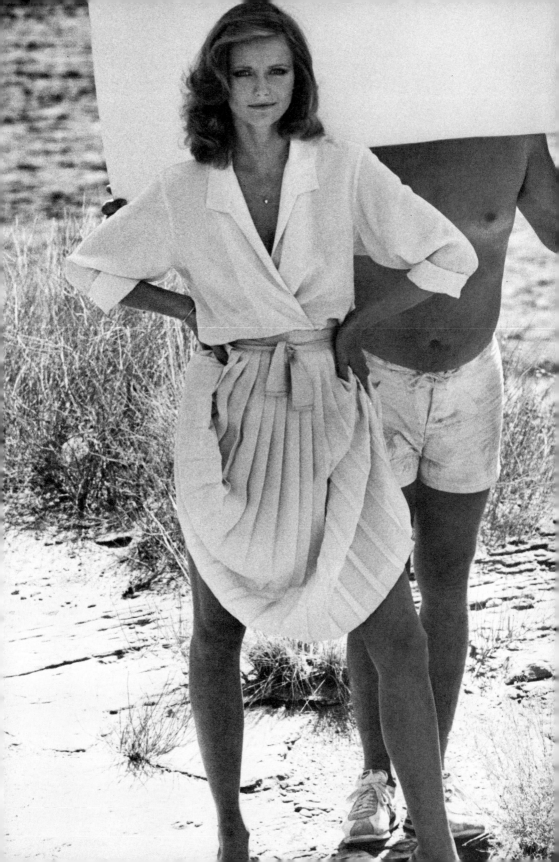

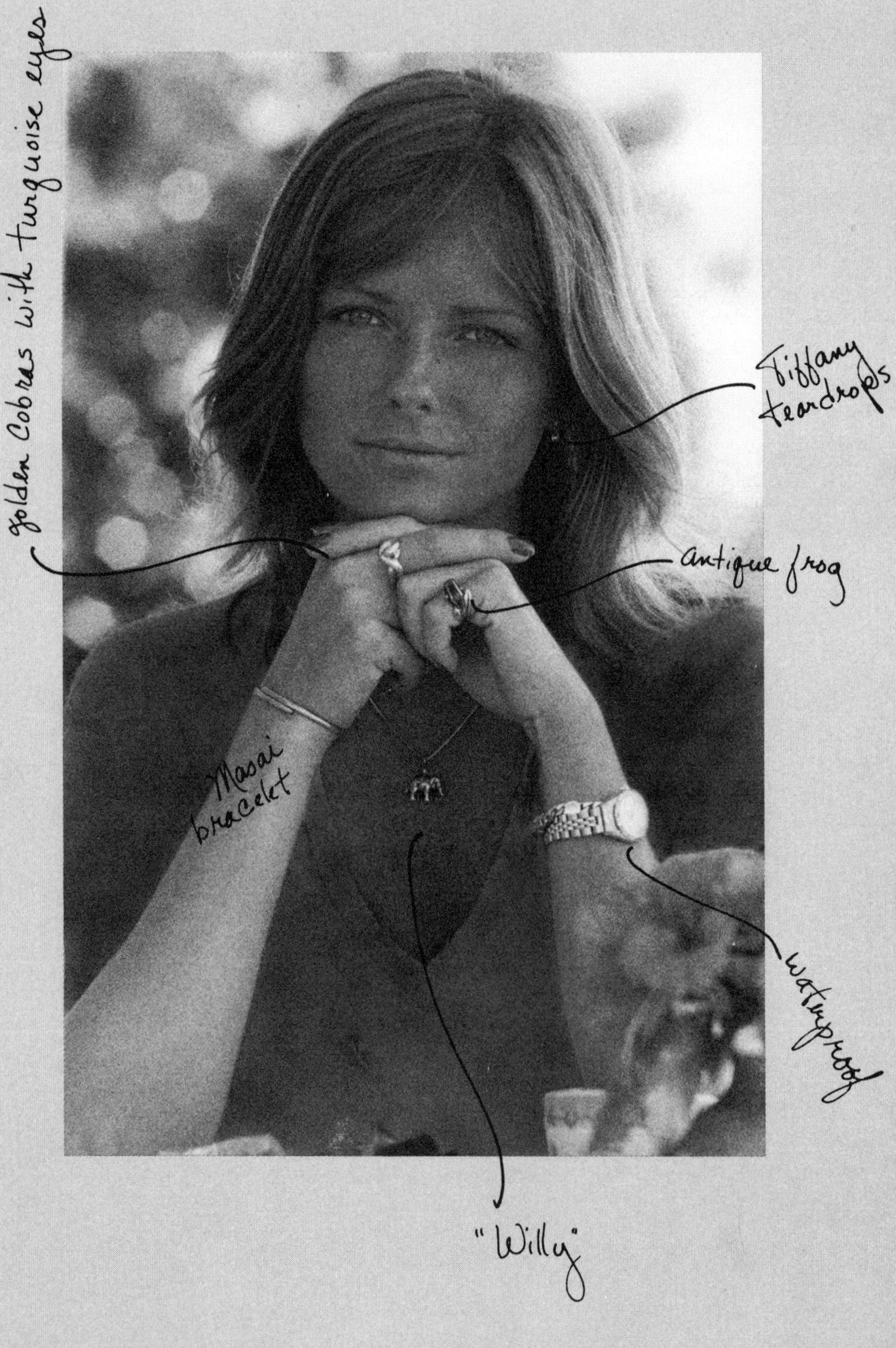

Golden Cobras with turquoise eyes

Tiffany teardrops

antique frog

Masai bracelt

waterproof

"Willy"

your legs the appearance of being shorter than they are. Stick with high heels in simple styles.

*Tall:* (C.T. answers to this one). Just relax and make the most of it, don't hide your height by slouching or wearing flat heels. I trafficked in my tallness even as a teenager; I wore high heels, I was proud to be tall. Tall women can get away with wearing almost anything, especially if they're on the thin side. I say "almost anything," because you'll surely want to stay away from long straight dresses in one color. Color contrasts in "separates," and vests, belts, and textured stockings will break up the long lines of your body.

*Short-waisted:* Avoid separates, and high-waisted pants, skirts, and dresses (they'll emphasize your waist). Tunics, vests, the blouson look, and loose-fitted clothes will all suit you, as well as dresses and skirts with a dropped or gathered waistline. A thin belt worn slightly below the waistband of a skirt or pants will give the illusion of a longer waist. And go for pants or skirts with a thin waistband.

*Long-waisted:* That's C.T., too, and I find it much more of an asset than a liability. You can easily wear skirts or pants with high waistbands. I confess that I don't even mind a dress with a waistband that rides up an inch or so more than normal.

## USE ACCESSORIES TO THE HILT

Anyone who's become skilled at taking outfits and creating a "look" knows how accessories can add that inspired personal touch without which you might as well have been dressed by a computer or a chart. Here are some tips on how to wear accessories.

### Jewelry

Days, I usually wear a snake ring with turquoise eyes, a green art-nouveau frog ring with ruby eyes, a gold elephant on a chain around my neck, an African bracelet, given to me by a Masai who in affection bent it so compellingly around my wrist I've never been able to get it off (not that I'd want to), a Rolex watch that I can get wet and bang around all I want without fear of breaking, and small diamond teardrop earrings. Occasionally I do take all these baubles and bangles off (except for the untakeable-off African bracelet) and put on a single large, heavy ivory bracelet. All my jewelry, as you can see, is highly personal—and also mythic, since it's connected in one way or another to

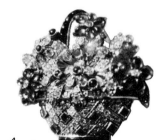

Cartier flower basket Circa 1890

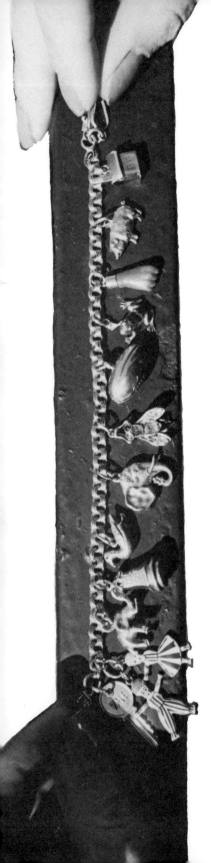

various people's pasts, and gives me a special feeling that goes way beyond the delimiting universe of fashionable appearance. For evenings, I have some wonderful antique watches and bracelets, some of which were given to me on nights when the wind kind of spreads your sails. Many people just pile on jewelry that has no real meaning for them except for what it all too obviously cost. I think your jewelry should represent some event or person in your life. I often remember a woman by the jewelry she wears; it tells me a lot more about her than how much money she has to spend on herself. Try using one or two pieces of jewelry to make a simple statement about yourself, or else wear one kind of jewelry, such as bracelets, earrings, rings, or special chains as your trademark. And then you'll wear the taste your trademark confers on you, not like a uniform, but like a badge.

### Belts

I must have the world's largest collection of belts. I'm convinced that a belt can do more than just about any other accessory to change the mood of an outfit. A rhinestone belt, worn with a pair of velvet jeans and a silk blouse, for example, can give a simple daytime outfit a glittering nighttime excitement. Double-wrap belts, rope belts, ties and cords can, one and all, change the line and look of whatever you have on. Use your imagination to create unusual and striking belts; try winding scarves or pieces of suede or cord from the yardage store around your waist. One of my most eccentric belt purchases never fails to make a hit. In St. Paul de Vence, over in the South of France, at a simple little leather goods store, I bought a belt whose buckle was made of the parts of a 1930s radio, so tune in to what I'm saying, okay?—and don't stick with the matching belt that comes with the outfit.

### Scarves and Hats

I seldom wear any of the many scarves I own. The best accessory is one you can put on and forget all about, and a scarf always seems to need redoing—at least mine does, I'm always having to put it back in place. If, however, you're stuck on scarves, practice wrapping and tieing them. But promise me you won't wear a scarf with a designer name on it—talk about insecurity. As the clever ad says, "When your own initials are enough."

There's one type of scarf I can't live without, though —the huge, oversized ones that come in soft cotton or silk. I travel with them and wear them as cover-ups on beaches or as robes in the blank, anonymous hotel rooms I sometimes have to stay in.

As for hats, I feel comfortable in them only if they're serving some purpose—otherwise I feel like I'm trying too hard. They can be fun, and even terribly flattering, but make sure you get the size right. If you have small features, go for the smaller brims—only people with large features can afford to wear wide or big-brimmed hats.

## COLOR AND TEXTURE

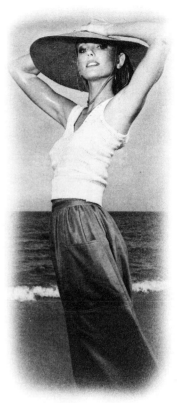

The color of the clothes a woman wears doesn't just bring out the tones of her skin and hair, it tells a lot about how she's feeling, what she's thinking, how friendly a face she presents to the world. Many women are timid when it comes to color; they buy clothes in the same shades over and over again, or else they wear colors in grimly limited combinations only. The foundation of a really great outfit is often an unexpected and surprising use of color, enhanced by the texture of the fabrics. Every color reflects differently on every face and, as you know, there are innumerable shades of the same basic color. You may discover that an off-shade of a color you always thought you hated looks fantastic on you and provides the perfect accent for some of your other garments as well. I've never liked the color yellow—it's always reminded me of kitchens and canaries (though don't get me wrong, I've got nothing against dishes and birds), but once I bought a mustard-colored blouse which turned out to go with everything I owned. I wore that blouse to death. So if you can't wear red, how about maroon; if you're wary of wearing purple, give mauve the old college try.

Don't play it safe by deciding that two colors are an automatic clash. How do you know till you've tried them together? When you buy a dress, hold it up to other dresses in the store. You may just spot that interesting color combination you've never before worn. Do the same with the clothes back in your closet.

As a general rule, bright colors work best as accents in blouses, sweaters, and scarves. One thing I always avoid is big bold prints too overpowering and, in the end, just plain boring. If muted colors appeal to you, select them in fabrics that have something a little out of the ordinary in the texture or weave. The pants and blouse of one of my most prized evening outfits come

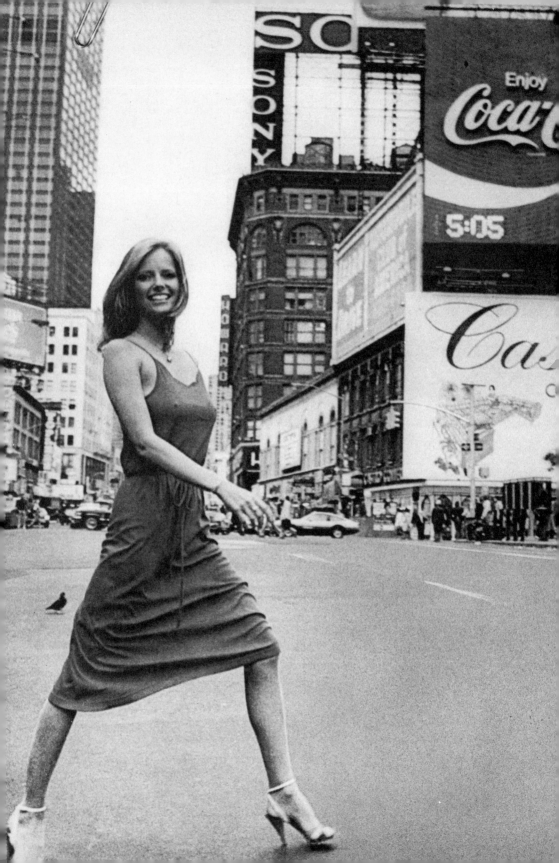

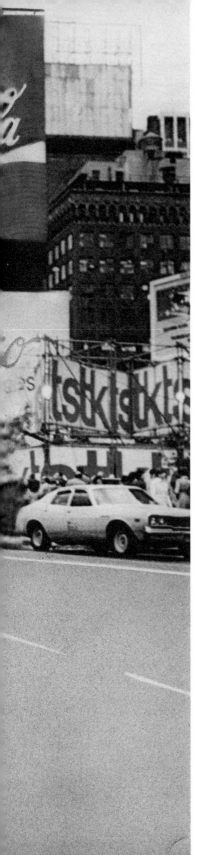

in lustrous beige satin—I call *that* a little out of the ordinary. The shininess of the satin takes the dull beige and makes it interesting. Sometimes I wear separates all in one color—like a dove-gray sweater with a dove-gray skirt, which I think of as an interesting non-combination.

## FEET, DO YOUR WORK!

When you're out shopping for shoes, it's sometimes hard to envision what kind will go best with the clothes you have. Moreover, when you get them home you often find they're a lot less comfortable than you imagined they'd be. I can't overemphasize the importance of wearing comfortable shoes, because when your feet hurt, they hurt and the whole evening is sacrificed.

I love high glittery sandals for evening. During the day I can't wear high heels because I do such a lot of walking. As one of my good friends said as she was about to run out to the store for groceries, "Feet, do your work!" and it wasn't high heels she had on. Did you know that if you wear high heels too often, you can throw your whole back out of alignment, and even distort the shape of your foot? When you buy high heels, make sure they're balanced correctly and can offer your foot the support it needs—otherwise you'll teeter-totter in them, a walking (sic) advertisement for the Old Comedy of Faults.

## CARE FOR YOUR CLOTHES AND SHOES

When a button pops or a zipper goes, repair the damage before you toss the garment in your closet or drawer. Or else what will happen is you'll forget all about it till you pull it out to wear, and then you'll be mighty disappointed. There's nothing that detracts from a well-groomed look more than unshined, run-down-at-the-heels shoes and boots. Keeping your shoes shined and in good repair also gives them a new lease on life—and a longer run for *your* money.

## MATERIALS FOR ALL SEASONS

Heavy cottons, rayons, ultra-suedes, velours, fine silks, corduroys, and many synthetics are comfortable in almost all seasons. Stretch your fashion budget and concentrate on long-lasting clothes that can be worn more than a couple of months a year. For warmth, simply add layers.

## CHOOSE YOUR OUTFITS IN ADVANCE

Don't wait till you're about to rush out the door to find the perfect outfit in your crowded closet. The afternoon or night before, try on your clothes in varying colors and textures. How does that silk skirt look with your favorite sweater? How well do your well-cut jeans go with that silk shirt? Consider wearing one silk shirt over another as kind of a jacket. Use your imagination. Ransack your drawers for accessories you haven't worn very much and put them together with your new clothes. When you've concocted a few exciting outfits, you won't have to ask before every big appointment or glamorous date, "What should I wear?" Oh me oh my!

## YOUR NOT-SO-CASUAL CASUAL LOOK

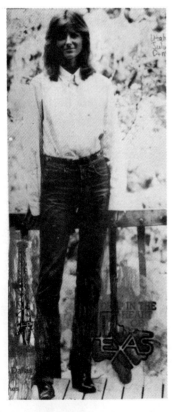

Audrey Hepburn knocked me out in *Two for the Road* wearing simply a pair of jeans, tennis shoes, and a T-shirt. I've always worn jeans and casual clothes—who hasn't?—but I discovered that there's a chasm deep and wide between a casual elegant look and a sloppy, thrown-together outfit that does nothing for me and less for the people who have to look at me. Never was this brought home to me more annihilatingly than the day I ran into my old friend Ali MacGraw outside Aida Thibiant's oasis of a salon in Beverly Hills. I had on tennis shoes, jeans, and a sweatshirt—an outfit I felt completely comfortable in and with—and one I always assumed I looked perfectly presentable in. Ali was wearing a cotton top, cotton pants, and sandals in magical shades of mauve and rose. The simplicity and clean lines of her outfit, combined with its sheer *practicality*, made me feel messy, which is about the last thing I like to feel. I kept my eyes glued to my dirty sneakers hoping she wouldn't notice what I was wearing (Fat chance!). That encounter led me to reconsider my casual look; by observing Ali, I learned that it was just as easy to put on an attractive casual outfit as it was to put on my sloppy clothes and dust-furred sneakers.

There's nothing cleaner, fresher than jeans and a cotton shirt, so long as the jeans fit and the shirt is pressed and well-tailored. This is another place where a single piece of jewelry can turn a neutral uniform into something stylish, another of the little creative "pushes" you can give to your look.

I've worked out some methods for dressing well and spending less time and money at it. They said it couldn't be done?

## DAY INTO NIGHT

Most of us are at work all day and don't have time to zip home and change before a cocktail party, dinner, or theater engagement. One good idea is to wear a simple skirt and a silk blouse to work and under the blouse a lacy camisole. Now unbutton the first two buttons of the blouse just as the evening begins. You might also keep a gold or rhinestone belt in your desk, and a small evening purse that's a snazzy nighttime alternative to your daytime pocketbook. Be sure to wear high-heeled sandals to work that day (or, once again, keep a pair in your desk). A velvet blazer can also turn a practical daytime look to one of instant evening elegance—garnished, perhaps, with a piece of your favorite jewelry. Well-tailored velvet jeans are always equally at home in the office and in a nightclub or discothèque.

## STOP 'N' SHOP IN YOUR FRIENDS' CLOSETS

Extend your wardrobe by trading and borrowing clothes. You may love a friend's fuscia blouse that it turns out *she hates*—and vice versa. I'm always borrowing and lending clothes. I had to go to Chicago on the spur of the moment a couple of years ago for a very important meeting, and found I had nothing really suitable in my overnight case. Instead of taking to the streets the first thing the next morning and shopping in a panic for something new, I borrowed a full, flattering pink dress from a friend. And I got the job!

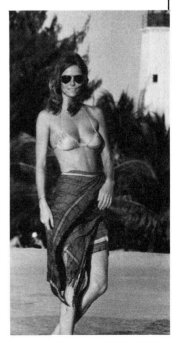

## TRY A DO-IT-YOURSELF KIKOY

When I was in Kenya filming my ABC-TV special, I "discovered" a fantastic thing called a "kikoy," which is a brightly colored piece of cotton fabric about 5' x 4'. I wrap it around my waist and tuck it in, and it makes a wonderful casual skirt, or I use it as a lounging outfit or a beach shawl. I often tuck it around my bikini bottom if I'm going straight from the beach to lunch. You can make your own kikoy by taking any scarf or large piece of fabric and simply wrapping it around your waist.

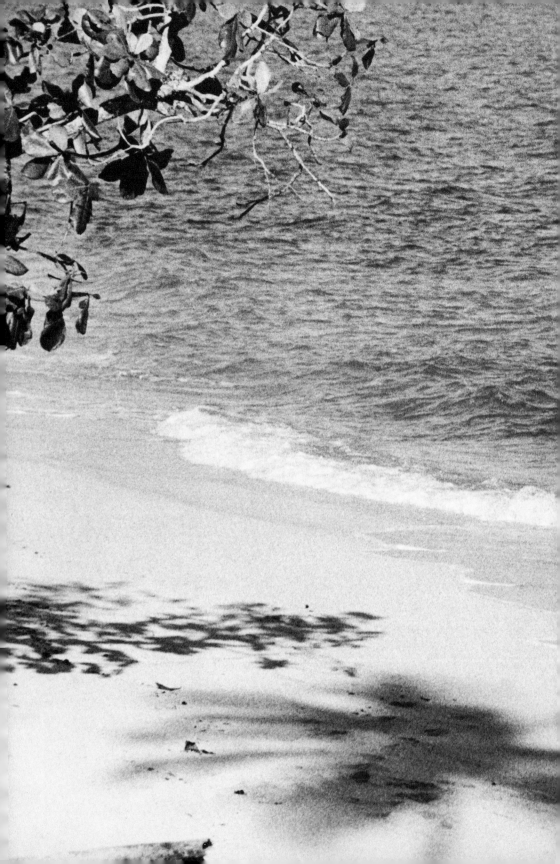

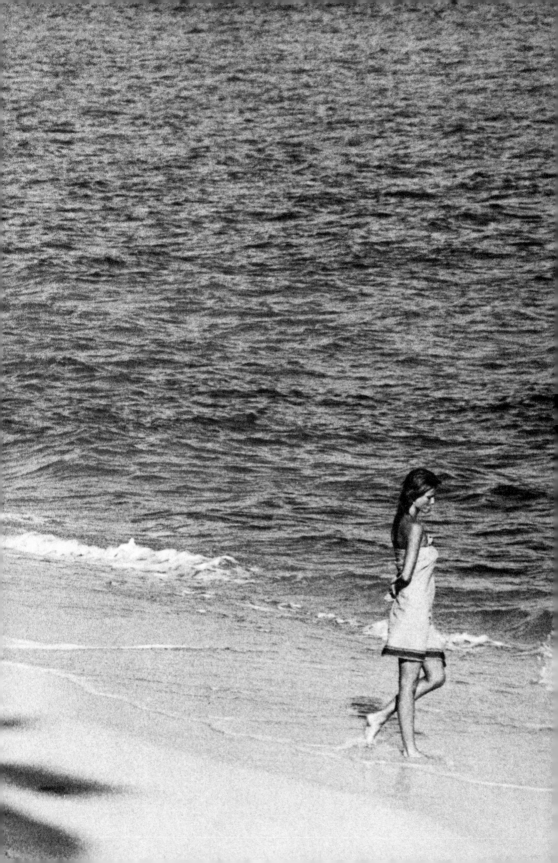

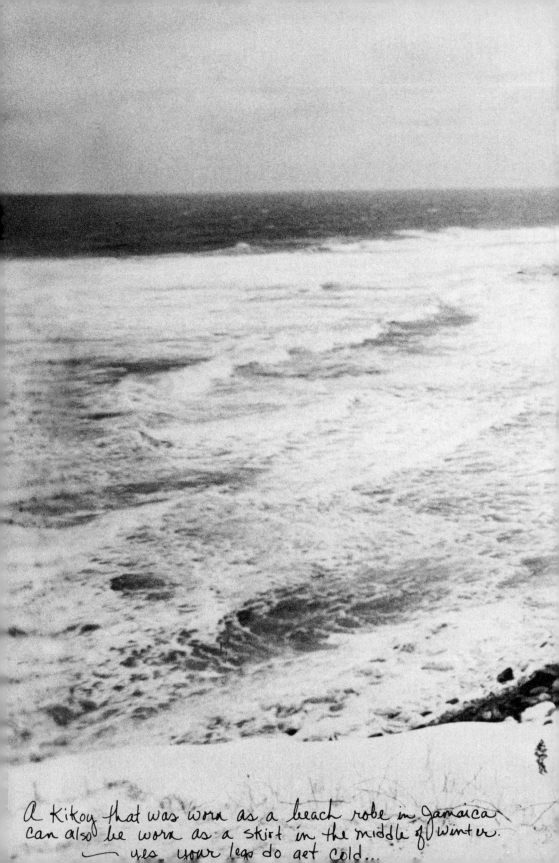

A kikoy that was worn as a beach robe in Jamaica
can also be worn as a skirt in the middle of winter.
— yes, your legs do get cold...

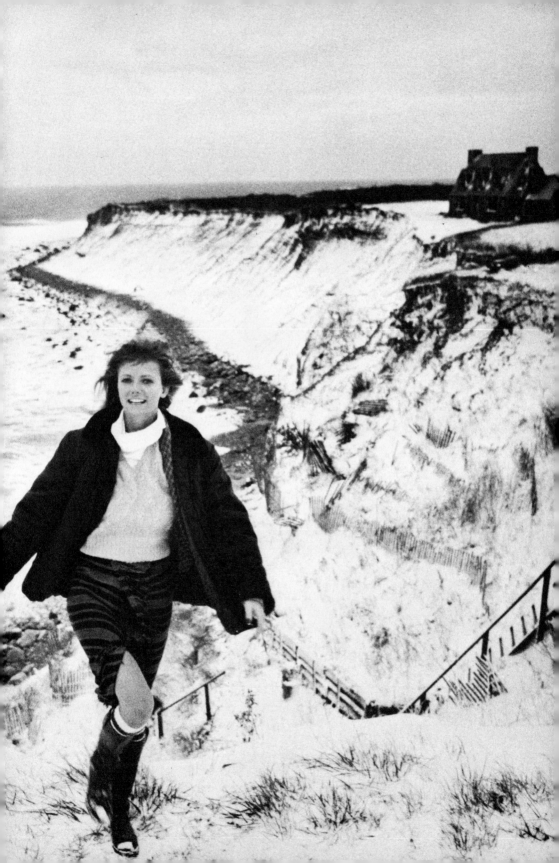

Because I travel so much, I've had to work out a real system for packing. I *always* pack three pairs of pants, one pair of jeans, two skirts, three sweaters, six blouses, and a couple of evening things. I make sure that most of the separates can be worn together. If I'm going to a cold place, I bring shirts, vests, and sweaters that can all be worn in layers for extra warmth. I always check out the climate before I go-go-go!

## MISTAKES PEOPLE MAKE

### Overdoing It

I've seen many well-known women, women with every possible advantage in life, pile on so much clothing and jewelry that all they succeed in doing is hiding the beauty or chic they would otherwise have in spades. This is just as bad as piling on too much makeup. The best-dressed woman knows that the most dramatic personal statement she can make is through simplicity. If you want to wear the latest hat, fine—just don't also wear the latest vest, the latest pants, the latest shoes, the latest stockings, the latest man's tie, and the latest stickpin. "Don't let your clothes walk in front of you," the saying goes.

### Shopping Madly Before a Special Occasion

I've made *this* mistake a lot myself. I was once invited to a fancy dress ball and told, "We're flying people in from Europe in private jets and everyone's going to be wearing one-of-a-kind designer dresses." I spent the entire day madly rushing around from shop to shop in a quest for the one dress that would take everyone's breath away. I couldn't find it. On an impulse I turned up wearing a very simple black evening dress—and you know what, I looked as good and chic as any of them. So don't knock yourself out shopping before a special occasion. You may find something spectacular all right—that will sit in your closet all the other 364 days of the year. Far better to wear an old favorite you feel completely at home in, completely yourself in (no, don't go in a "kikoy").

### Buying a Coat First

First of all, don't buy a coat before assembling your wardrobe. And when you do buy, buy one that fits over your jackets and sweaters and is slightly longer than your skirts and dresses. Choose a model that has good lines and a great fabric, but don't go overboard and buy a purple coat with tangerine flowers—pick a shade that has staying power.

### Looking Inappropriate

No matter how beautiful your outfit is, you'll feel pretty silly in it if it's not appropriate to the occasion. A few months ago I appeared at a party in a soft wool skirt, cotton blouse, high heels, and bow tie. Everyone else there was dressed to kill—it was a big bow-wow party—in silk and satin evening clothes. I knew I looked good but I felt almost criminally out of place, so naturally I didn't enjoy the evening—for one thing, I couldn't quite bring myself to hit the dance floor out there among all the sleek silhouettes under the twinkling lights and toy balloons. Take the trouble to phone your hostess and find out beforehand what kind of dress to wear.

### Buying Pre-Selected Outfits

Don't blindly buy a skirt or pants with a top or vest manufactured to go with it. These "perfectly matching" outfits can be altogether perfectly depressing and unimaginative and show that you *prefer* running in a pack. There may be safety in numbers, but there isn't much style. Trust yourself a little and choose an outfit that reflects *your* taste. Mixin' and minglin' is always more fun than blindly matchin'.

### Fretting Over Minuscule Wrinkles and Spots

We Americans are much too involved with ironing and Clorox. Many women reject beautiful fabrics out of the misplaced fear that they won't have time to keep them perfectly pressed. They worry too much about wrinkles and spots too tiny for a naked eye to see. Of course, keep your clothes clean, but don't relinquish quality for drip-dry, non-wrinkle polyester.

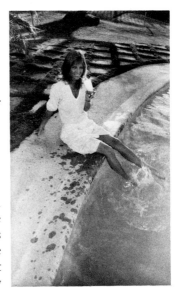

### Underestimating the Importance of Your Clothes

Whether you like it or not, you are going to be judged partly by how you dress. Psychologists say that people who pay absolutely no attention to their wardrobes may be suffering from a poor self-image, and that the reason they wear sloppy or anonymous clothes is that they subconsciously long to advertise the negative way they feel about themselves; some go so far as to wear clothes *calculated* to diminish their sex appeal and keep them secure in the background—they're that afraid to project themselves. If you're totally indifferent to clothes and all your life have been claiming you just couldn't care less, there are more important things to worry about, maybe you should ask yourself a very uncomfortable question—"Why?"

Mind you, I'm not saying that I think clothes are the be-all and end-all or even the most all-all-all of them all. Everything in its place. Shopping can be frustrating, vexing, maddening. But the result is often worth the trouble. It was no less august a figure than Emerson who wrote: "the lady declared that the sense of being perfectly well-dressed gives a feeling of inner tranquility which religion is powerless to bestow."

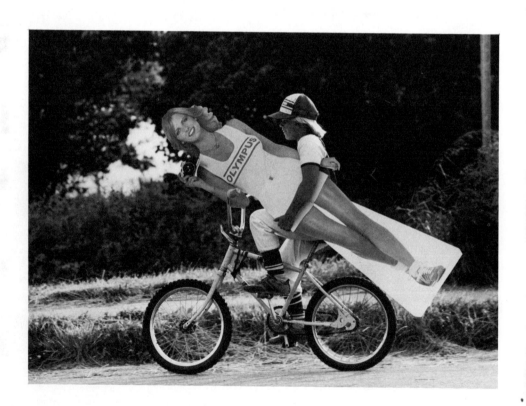

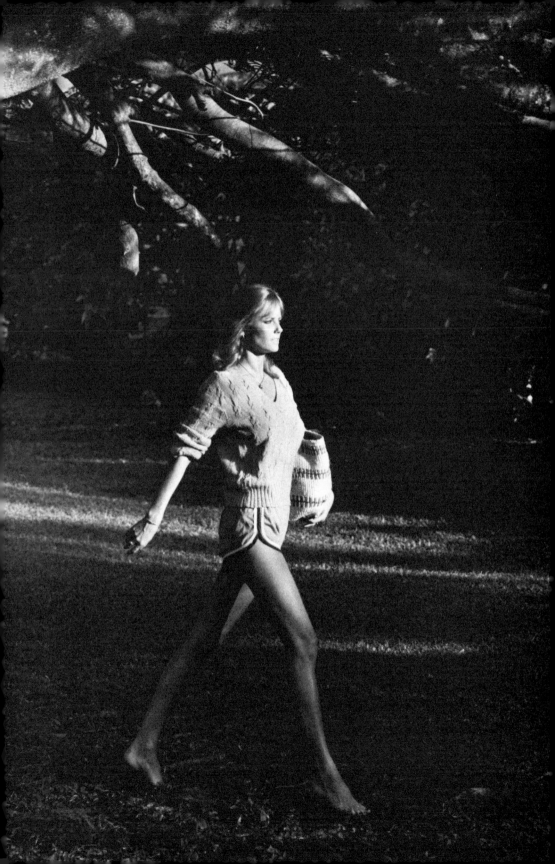

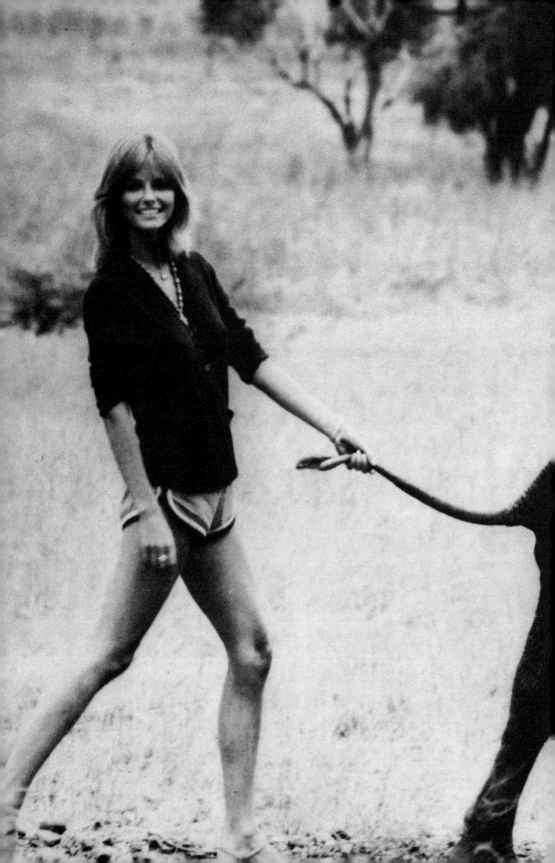

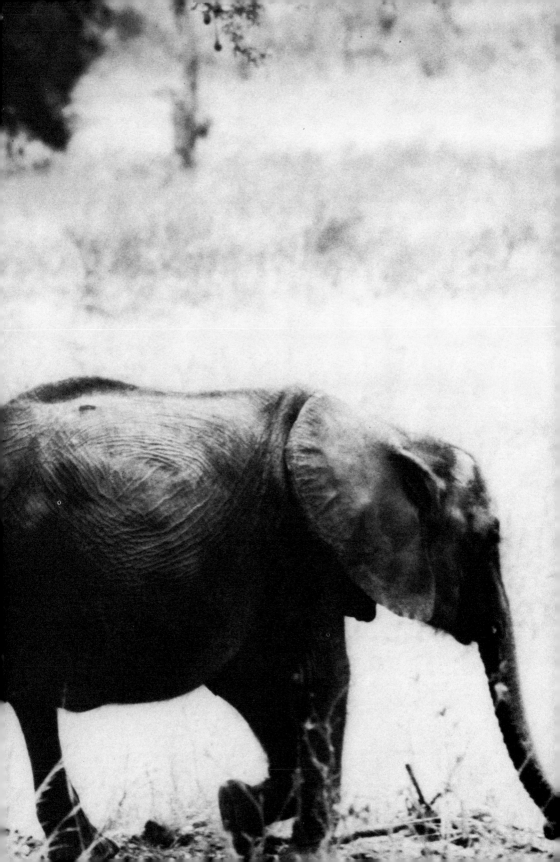

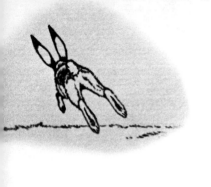

# 9

# Odds & Ends: You're Only as Good as the Finishing Touches

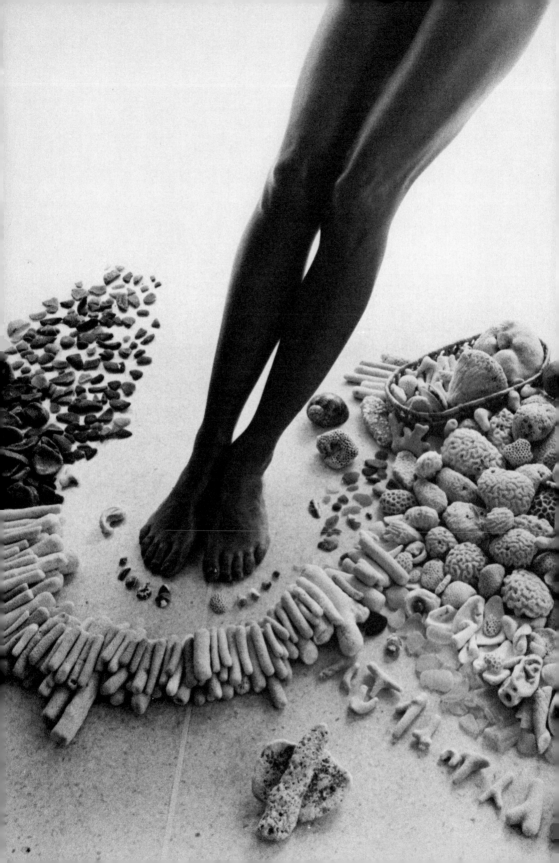

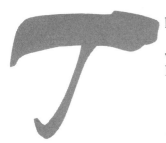

he quality called attractiveness is a function of the whole person; you can't be, like the curate's egg, only "good in places." You must be aware of all parts of your body: how your shoulders sit, your smile, fidgeting hands and feet, your fragrance, and—the sum and extension of all these parts—your attitude, which is, after all, the image of your image. Neglect the "invisible" basics of grooming and health care and they won't stay invisible for long; they will emerge with a force all the greater for their suppression and ultimately sabotage whatever efforts you've made with your wardrobe, makeup, and hair.

Here are the things I've learned to watch out for when it comes time to polish up my appearance.

## THE IMPORTANCE OF STANDING STRAIGHT

All through junior high I hated dancing class because I was so much taller than all the boys. Back then, those extra inches felt like miles. Fortunately I had a mother who encouraged me to take pride in the fact that I was a tall girl, and thanks to her, I learned to stand straight, and bypassed the tall girl's slump: the rounded shoulders and curved back that many short girls also manage to saddle themselves with. Today it feels even better than it did then to be tall, and when I really want to get way up there I put on my high-heeled gold sandals and tower over everyone, "taller than the tallest building!"

Good posture has certainly been a big plus in all my modeling jobs. (Bad posture can disqualify an aspiring model on the spot.) Many girls seem to have completely forgotten how to walk normally. And that's a great shame, for aside from doing a lot for any outfit, good bearing makes *you* look better—slimmer and more assuming, someone with real "presence." If you're apt to become nervous when you enter a room, straighten those shoulders, hold your head up, and move on in, as if the room belongs to you. Good posture can give the lie to whatever self-doubts might be consuming you in your personal life and holding you back in your career.

Too many people these days don't have the slightest awareness of the way they sit and stand. After you've

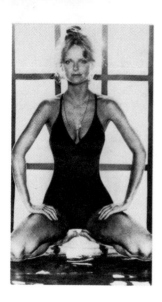

answered the following questions, you should have a pretty good idea as to just how good your posture is.

■ *Are your shoulders sometimes tense and all hunched forward?*

■ *Does your chin jut out? Or is it tucked down and pushed back? Or does it tilt up?*

■ *Is the part of your back just below your neck straight or slightly curved?*

■ *Is there an S-shaped curve in the small of your back?*

■ *Do you always have a pot belly, no matter how thin you are?*

If you answered yes to any one of these questions, the chances are you did to all of them—because poor posture has a chain-link effect on how your body looks. Tense, hunched shoulders make your neck tense, which in turn gives your head a slightly lopsided look. And, if your shoulders and head aren't held in a straight line, your back won't be straight, either. And a curve in the small of the back almost always means there's going to be a pot belly out there somewhere. Or, as the poet might have put it, if a pot belly is here, can a curve in the small of the back be far behind? Seriously, you run a big risk of having every part of your body become slightly deformed, and these deformities can become permanent with time: the old lady's hump is the fearful legacy of her lifelong habit of slumping. And did you know that really bad posture can cause back pain and headaches as well as cramp the style of the lungs (and the style of the lungs, in case you didn't know, is a little function called breathing!). You owe it to yourself to stand up straight—that is, unless you want to look like a hovel and feel like one. Don't let bad posture become a metaphor for your whole life.

## HOW TO DEVELOP GOOD POSTURE

### Exercise

It shouldn't come as any great revelation that women who've been doing ballet for years have better posture than other women. Not every woman can (do ballet), but there are many other kinds of exercise that not only make you conscious of the way you stand, but develop the muscles that hold your body up: swimming, yoga, calisthenics, and *any* kind of dance training will all strengthen your supporting muscles as well as make you fully aware of how they work.

### Vigilance

Even though I have fairly good posture, I make a point of checking it out in the mirror: Are my shoulders back and down? Am I holding my stomach up and in? Are my head and neck poised directly on top of the spine? If you make a posture check at specific times every day, you'll begin to see your bad habits standing out in bold relief. And knowledge of them is the first step toward correcting them. Check your posture when you're sitting down, too. If you have a desk-oriented job, try keeping your feet on the ground, your chin in, and your back straight. By sitting straight when you're at your desk, you'll feel less tired when your workday is over.

### Posture Exercises

Close your eyes and imagine that someone is pulling you up by a string attached to your head. Unless you're John the Baptist, you should be able to feel your whole body lengthen and straighten.

Now lie on the floor on your back and bend your knees. Press your whole back, and also the back of your neck, right into the floor. Now slowly, slowly straighten your legs, continuing to press your back into the floor.

Ahhh . . . !

## FLASH THE WHITE TEETH OF THE HAPPY GIRL

I was shocked when I read recently that roughly one half of all Americans don't bother to visit a dentist even once a year. God! I always have my teeth checked and cleaned at least twice a year.

Many people lose their teeth and, worse, become the victims of gum disease: the guaranteed result of improper brushing and flossing. Achieving and maintaining good dental hygiene require almost as much in the way of time and attention as your makeup application does. But it's worth it, since there is nothing more costly, inconvenient, frightening, and painful than the elaborate procedures necessary to restore your teeth and gums. It's not called tooth "decay" for nothing: they go downhill fast, once they begin to go, and down you go along with them, down into "the country of the general lost freshness." So practice these four cardinal rules and save your teeth—and your beautiful smile.

### 1. Sugar

Like the rest of your body, your teeth and gums need a varied, nutritious diet. It's the same foods that make you fat that destroy your teeth. And the main enemy, an unnatural enemy if there ever was one, is *sugar*. It joins with the bacteria in your mouth to form acids and plaque that eat your teeth and gums away. If you just can't help yourself and you do eat sugar, then get it out of your mouth as fast as you can. And eat a lot of crunchy, fibrous raw fruits and vegetables, which help clean your teeth.

### 2. Brushing

Make sure you get the brush as close to the gumline as possible, and brush *all* the surfaces of your teeth. Use a fluoride toothpaste, but stay away from special teeth whiteners, which are said to be too harsh on the enamel. For a special whitening treatment, brush once a week with baking soda, which makes for a good old-fashioned, slightly abrasive toothpaste, in addition to your regular brushing. Brush twice a day—and always before bedtime, because bacteria remains longest in the mouth—doing its nasty work—while you're fast asleep.

### 3. Flossing

Brushing is not enough! To prevent the dreaded plaque from building up on your teeth, you must use dental floss. Your toothbrush alone cannot possibly remove food particles from between the teeth and close to the gums. Flossing is no joke: it prevents gum disease more effectively than any other form of home dental care.

### 4. See Your Dentist

Don't see your dentist only when you have a toothache, because by then you're already in trouble. Most tooth decay and gum erosion begin with no betrayal of discomfort. A good and easy way to practice preventive dental care is simply to have minor work done on a regular basis. If your home dental care habits are not what they should be, then by all means have your

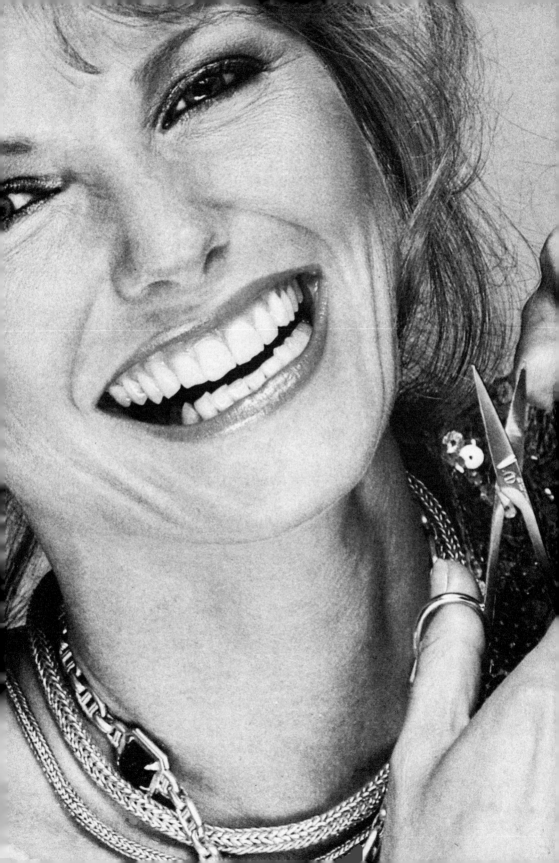

teeth professionally cleaned at least a couple of times a year.

## FINGERNAIL POWER

A model's hands are one of the most pliant, expressive, and revealing parts of her body. I'm often surprised how my hands stand out in photographs, and how the gestures I make with them add or detract from the general picture. It goes without saying that there is no way your hands can be appealing if your fingernails are not well-groomed. A lot of women seem to be under the unfortunate impression that "well-groomed" means long, red nails (the better to maul you with, my dear?). I was once the victim of this misconception myself. When I stopped working and didn't have all that much to do with myself, I became a slave to nail polish. It sounds like a joke, but believe me, it wasn't. Every week I had a manicure, and if one of my holier-than-thou nails so much as chipped or cracked or—heaven forbid—actually broke, I dashed back to the body shop for repairs. My nails finally got so long I couldn't zip my zippers or button my buttons by myself—I mean, I might just as well have been on a life-support system. As soon as I got out of the house and went back to work, I dispensed with the nail routine.

There's no question that perfectly manicured, painted nails are fun for all the world to see. Beyond that, though, they raise some troubling questions, since they obviously mean you're not doing anything very strenuous or life-enhancing, like gardening or sailing. I think a good solution is a short, well-groomed nail, clean and glossy, coated with a clear polish, which can be every bit as beautiful as a long, red talon and which has the added advantage of making your hands look *capable* and *natural*.

### The Ten-Minute All-Natural Mini-Manicure!

Flash! Here's a five-step manicure that takes only minutes.

1. Remove your old polish.
2. Gently push your cuticles back with an orangewood stick, covered with cotton.
3. File with a nail file or emery board in one direction only. Round the corners, but don't file the sides (this will make your nails weak). Try not to cut your nails with scissors (this will make them brittle) or to

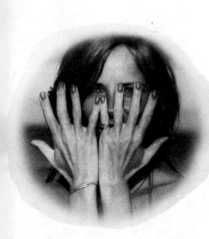

file after a nail has been immersed in water and is soft and fragile.

4. Buff your nails with a natural hide buffer to give them a natural shine. Buffing also improves the circulation of the nail. (For a maxi-mini-manicure, stop here! Do not proceed to 5.)

5. Apply a clear polish. If you like a bright polish, apply a base coat of clear polish first. Different polishes wear off at different rates. You'll just have to experiment till you find one that stays on.

## MISTAKES PEOPLE MAKE

### Using a Cuticle Clipper

Cutting your cuticle will only make it big and tough, which is probably not what you had in mind. So always push your cuticle back, then just leave it alone. Treat any ragged cuticles with a cuticle cream. To soften your cuticles and prevent rough, red hands, rub Vaseline into your entire hand; if you want to go to extremes, wear white gloves to bed.

### Removing Polish Too Often

When a nail chips, instead of removing all your nail polish (this will dry the nail), just add a touch-up coat.

### The Gelatin-Cocktail-Hour Syndrome

You can drink a thousand and one unflavored gelatin cocktails and still they will not make your nails grow longer. Polish actually does more to harden and protect your nails than anything you could ever eat. (A protein-rich diet, however, is important for both hair and nails, which are composed of a protein substance.) If you want long nails and, no matter how hard you try, you just can't seem to grow them, ask your manicurist to wrap them in a paper shield to protect the growing nail.

### Be Kind to Your Fingers

If you pull at hangnails, bite your fingernails, or jam your fingers into a jammed-up handbag, you have some bad habits to overcome. Remember, "Don't make frazzled nails the mirror of frazzled nerves."

One's feet are usually visible only at intimate moments (many men by the way, find a beautiful foot a real turn-on) or at the beach. Unlike your hands, your feet have limited powers of expression (this side of kicking!), and to look good, they must be pampered. I rub the rough, dry areas of my feet with a pumice stone and try not to overlook my feet when I'm applying lotion to my body. A painted, well-groomed toenail is a must in an open-toed sandal. Clip your toenails to a smooth oval, then smooth the rough edges with a file, and separate your toes with cotton pads before you apply the enamel so it won't smudge.

Don't sacrifice your feet to good-looking, but constricting—even killing—shoes. They'll just give you corns, bunions, and other unsightly ailments. If you've already gone and bought a pair of fabulously expensive and unbelievably uncomfortable high heels, I guess you're going to feel you have to wear them just to get your money's worth—but wear them for a couple of hours at a time only! The agonies of having aching feet, along with the tiresome grumbling you're bound to do, will eventually show up graven on your face. Try soaking your feet in very hot water and then plunging them into a cold bath. In summer, when they're apt to get overheated, spray your feet with a light cologne; the alcohol will cool them off.

## THE SWEET SMELL OF . . . YOU!

The perfume you wear creates an aura, like a sub-light; lingers in the air, and in the memories of those you come into contact with. I always wear perfume. My favorites are Oscar de la Renta, Madame de Balmain, and Chanel #5. I usually finish a bottle of one of these before I switch my allegiance to another, because it's nice to identify with a single perfume for a while, let it mark a time in your life, the time of your time which if you're lucky may even be the time *of* your life.

Back in my salad days, I once took the advice of a fashion magazine and set my hair with perfume before a party. When the curlers came out the scent hung over me like a cloud, like a reproach that reeked. Too much perfume is much worse than none. Any insistent odor can ruin an appetite, yours and others'. A touch of scent behind the ears, a dab on the neck or along the torso, is far more provocative than an envel-

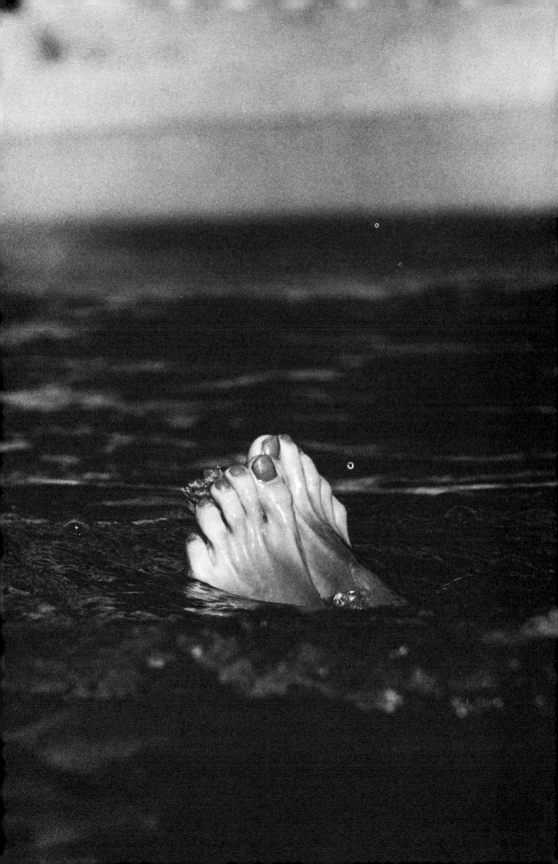

oping fog of the stuff. For a very light scent, spray your favorite perfume into the air and walk through the shower of tiny droplets.

### Selecting a Scent

Don't choose perfumes just because they're new or "different," or have seductive names, or smell good on your friends. Body chemistry very subtly changes the fragrance of perfume; also, the longer you keep it on, the more it changes. The seasons also have an effect on scent, so when it's hot, you should use a light fragrance in preference to a heavy, exotic one. By the same token, it's a good idea not to wear perfume in the sun—some of the ingredients can spot your skin when exposed to ultraviolet rays.

### Instead of Perfume, What?

Use a few drops of good bath oil, that's what. Bath oil scents are often quite heady and, used as a substitute for perfume, make your bath all the sweeter.

A great-smelling soap is an inexpensive way to smell fresh. And use a bar of it, left in its wrapper, to scent your lingerie drawer. For a really spicy fragrance—if you want him to feel that old, warm, spicy breeze blowing—switch to a man's cologne.

## SLEEP, BEAUTIFUL SLEEP

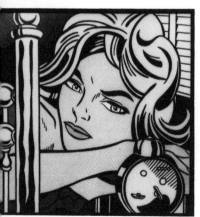

"Blonde Waiting"
Roy Lichtenstein—1964

Lack of sleep not only makes you look a bit out of it, whatever "it" is, but also fosters a sort of worm's-eye view of the world that doesn't exactly help either the world or you. Irritation, lethargy, and lassitude are some of the more attractive results of insomnia. Each of us requires a different number of hours of sleep, "sleep that knits up the ravelled sleeve of care," and our requirements change as we get older. Most of us, for example, need more sleep during periods of stress, and less when we're doing something we enjoy.

Stress keeps us from falling asleep easily. When I'm on the road and working hard, or socially overindulging myself, or not getting enough exercise, it's sometimes a real struggle for me to get the sleep my body needs. I've had to work up a few tricks and routines to get by on.

### C.T.'s Never-Say-Die Cures for Insomnia

Every night before I lay me down to sleep, I wash my face, straighten my apartment up, and close all the doors, even the closets. (Everybody has some little neurosis about the sleeping ritual and mine is closing all the doors. Indulge yourself!) The point I want to make is that if you follow some regular bedtime pattern, your psyche will come to associate it with deep slumber.

And how about a glass of milk before bedtime? It contains a sleep-inducing amino acid called "tryptophan," that's especially helpful if you suffer from acid indigestion. If you don't like your milk cold, heat it with a quarter teaspoon of vanilla and add a teaspoon of honey—it's yummy. Calcium tablets also are a great natural sleeping pill. Even a little old aspirin can relax your muscles and help you fall asleep. Avoid barbiturates at any and all costs: they can be addictive and, gobbled in large doses, can actually *prevent* you from getting to sleep (and if and when you do, you may have the foulest nightmares). On the very few occasions when I've resorted to sleeping pills, I've paid the high price of being too groggy the next morning to function effectively, to perform at the top of the tent, so to speak (so *not* to speak?).

Just before turning in, I organize the following day in my mind, and then write down all my appointments. I think through the problems that are preying on me so that half-baked plans and nagging worries can't keep me awake and fretful. If I find my mind getting stuck on all my problems while I'm trying to find sleep, I concentrate on one thing at a time, instead of letting everything gang up on me.

I imagine—or, depending on the weather outside my windowpane, fantasize—that I'm lying on a beach in the unwavering heat of noon, so that my body is infused with that peaceful, somnolent feeling born of sun and sea and good clean air. Sometimes I imagine —or, again, fantasize—that someone is rocking me slowly in a hammock. Another trick I have for defeating, or at least subduing, tension: I relax one part of my body at a time—toes, feet, ankles, calves—right on up to my head, which is often in the clouds because my castle's in the sky. It works! And why shouldn't it? Because what is sleep if not a question of mind over matter? If my plane lands in New York from Los Angeles at night, I adjust to East Coast time simply by telling myself, "It's midnight and time for bed!" instead of panicking, "How will I ever get to sleep?" Thinking makes it so!

I keep a "dream pad" beside my bed, and every morning I write down whatever I can remember from the night before. God, the things you can learn about yourself! Looking forward to dreaming can be an incentive to get to sleep.

If you really, really can't sleep, don't surrender to the misery of tossing and turning. Don't just lie there, *do* something! Get up, for a start. How about a few stretching exercises? There's always the TV, or a good book. Try to relax. You have a lot at stake: your peace of mind.

### Exercise: Again and Then Again!

At the risk of becoming the nag of all time: now *is* the time and this *is* the place to reiterate that few people who exercise regularly suffer from insomnia. Exercise rids your muscles of the tension that keeps you awake.

### Create a Room That's Good to Sleep in

A cold room begets a cold, shivering sleep. I painted mine a warm, relaxing color and I sleep well, with all my plants and books and thoughts and things around. A humidifier helps keep the lining of my nose and throat from drying out, and the hum, surprisingly, is soothing. Make sure your mattress is firm and that the bed board under the mattress is three-quarters of an inch thick. This also makes for both a comfortable night and a strong back. Despite the dozens of decorative pillows you see piled up in magazine layouts of bedrooms, don't ever sleep on more than one, because if your neck gets over-elevated, it may be stiff in the morning—and for several days running. And a stiff neck is not the finishing touch you want. You want to wake up sweetened by your good night's sleep—and holding in your hand the key to all life's secret little graces.

But alas, the knowledge of how to make yourself attractive doesn't arrive in a dream, at least not in any dream I know of.

> To be born woman is to know—
> Although they do not talk of it at school—
> That we must labour to be beautiful.
> —W. B. Yeats, "Adam's Curse"

Oh, it may be a struggle, it may even be a fight, but to quote Colette again, "It is the fight itself that keeps you young."

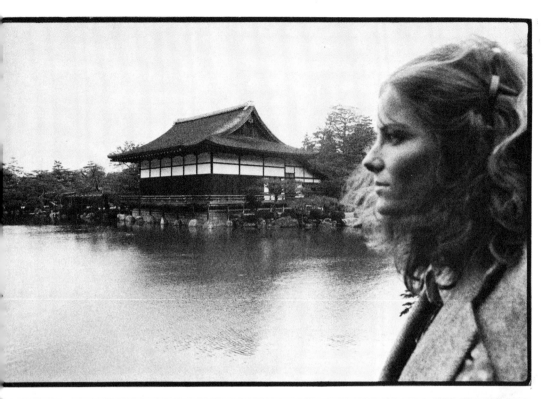

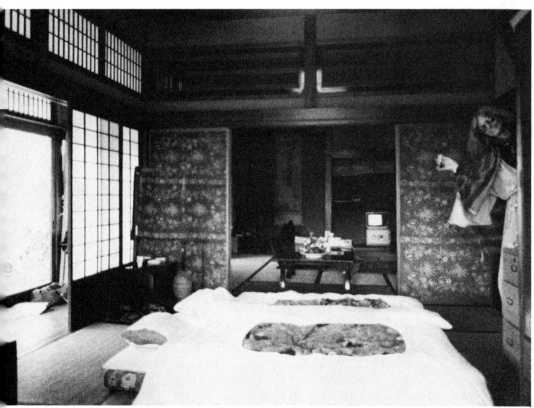

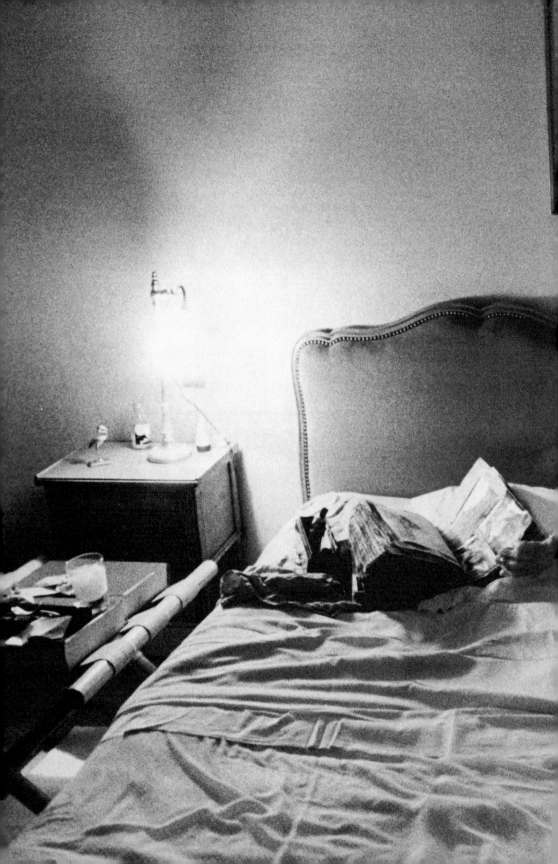

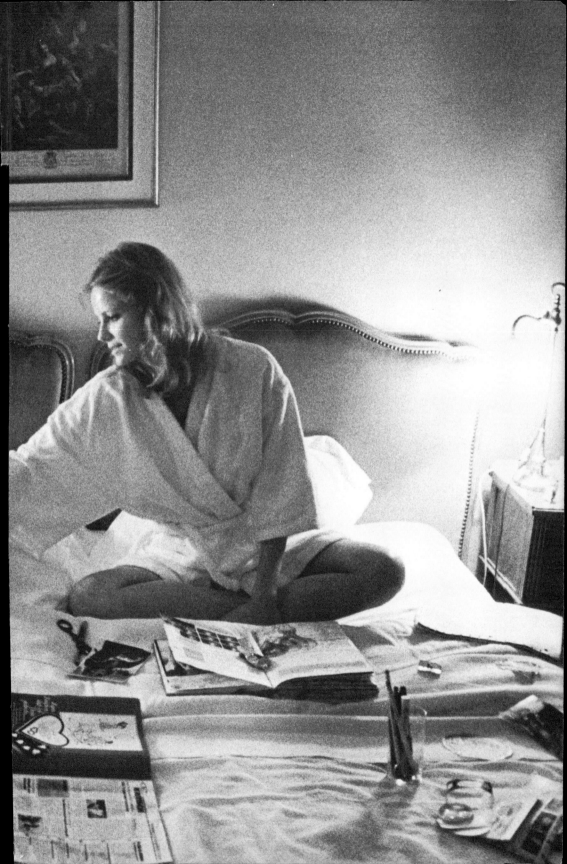

Photographs are reproduced by the kind permission of the following: